NUTRITION AND DIET RESEARCH PROGRESS

DIETARY SUPPLEMENTS: WHAT SENIORS NEED TO KNOW

NUTRITION AND DIET RESEARCH PROGRESS

Additional books in this series can be found on Nova's website under the Series tab.

Additional E-books in this series can be found on Nova's website under the E-books tab.

AGING ISSUES, HEALTH AND FINANCIAL ALTERNATIVES

Additional books in this series can be found on Nova's website under the Series tab.

Additional E-books in this series can be found on Nova's website under the E-books tab.

NUTRITION AND DIET RESEARCH PROGRESS

DIETARY SUPPLEMENTS: WHAT SENIORS NEED TO KNOW

THOMAS H. FELTON

EDITOR

Nova Science Publishers, Inc.

New York

For permission to use material from this book please contact us:
Telephone 631-231-7269; Fax 631-231-8175
Web Site: http://www.novapublishers.com

NOTICE TO THE READER

LIBRARY OF CONGRESS CATALOGING-IN-PUBLICATION DATA

Dietary supplements : what seniors need to know / editor, Thomas H. Felton.
p. ; cm.
Includes bibliographical references and index.
ISBN 978-1-61761-285-5 (hardcover)
1. Dietary supplements--United States. 2. Older people--Nutrition--United States. I. Felton, Thomas H.
[DNLM: 1. Dietary Supplements--United States. 2. Aged--United States. 3. Consumer Product Safety--United States. QU 145.5]
RM258.5.D55 2010
613.2'6--dc22
2010027281

Published by Nova Science Publishers, Inc. † New York

CONTENTS

PREFACE

Dietary supplements have become a multi-billion dollar industry. In 2006, Americans reportedly spent $23 billion on herbal and specialty supplements, which is almost half the amount they spent on prescription drugs. However, several consumer safety issues arise with these products. Because dietary supplements are available over-the-counter, consumers sometimes take them in addition to, or even as a replacement for, other prescription medication or drugs without consulting their doctors or receiving notification of potentially harmful interactions. This book examines and addresses concerns that have arisen over whether the marketing and manufacturing of these products meet the standards that American consumers deserve.

Chapter 1- . The use of dietary supplements, which can take the form of vitamins, minerals, fiber, or other nutritional products, has grown substantially over the past few decades. Recent surveys indicate that at least 40 percent of American adults consume these products, many of which can serve as a valuable and nutritional addition to daily diets. Today we will address concerns that have arisen over whether the marketing and manufacturing of these products meet the standards that American consumers deserve.

Dietary supplements have become a multi-billion dollar industry. In 2006, Americans reportedly spent $23 billion on herbal and specialty supplements, which is almost half the amount they spent on prescription drugs. However, several consumer safety issues arise with these products. Because dietary supplements are available overthe-counter, consumers sometimes take them in addition to, or even as a replacement for, other prescription medication or drugs without consulting their doctors or receiving notification of potentially harmful interactions.

Chapter 2- Recent studies have shown that use of herbal dietary supplements—chamomile, echinacea, garlic, ginkgo biloba, and ginseng—by the elderly within the United States has increased substantially. Sellers, such as retail stores, Web sites, and distributors, often claim these supplements help improve memory, circulation, and other bodily functions. GAO was asked to determine (1) whether sellers of herbal dietary supplements are using deceptive or questionable marketing practices and (2) whether selected herbal dietary supplements are contaminated with harmful substances.

To conduct this investigation, GAO investigated a nonrepresentative selection of 22 storefront and mail-order retailers of herbal dietary supplements. Posing as elderly consumers, GAO investigators asked sales staff (by phone and in person) at each retailer a series of questions regarding herbal dietary supplements. GAO also reviewed written marketing language used on approximately 30 retail Web sites. Claims were evaluated against recognized scientific research published by the National Institutes of Health (NIH) and the Food and Drug Administration (FDA). GAO also had an accredited lab test 40 unique popular single-ingredient herbal dietary supplements for the presence of lead, arsenic, mercury, cadmium, organichlorine pesticides, and organophosphorous pesticides.

Chapter 3- A recent survey of people who receive our free e-newsletter revealed that that *among those aged 65 and older, 32% use 10 or more supplements daily* (Reference 1).

A senior citizen in a vitamin store is a bit like a kid a candy store. However, while the FDA recommends a strict limit on lead contamination in candy, it has not set a limit for supplements. Our tests show that this policy has created a " buyer beware" situation.

Chapter 4- Consumers and seniors turn to dietary supplements because they think these products will promote health and wellness. They also generally assume that such products are safe for their intended use, and would not be permitted to be sold by the federal government if they were unsafe or posed unreasonable risks to consumers. Unfortunately, in this research and reporting, we have found some very profound and troubling gaps in the system we have today to assure supplement safety. While many dietary supplements, including most vitamins and minerals taken within recommended limits, are generally safe and can have important health benefits for consumers, there is a significant and growing number of highly questionable products that would probably not be allowed on the market if they were subject to rigorous pre-market safety testing.

Chapter 5- The Council for Responsible Nutrition (CRN) appreciates this opportunity to provide testimony to the Senate Special Committee on Aging on behalf of the dietary supplement industry to reassure you and your colleagues, your constituents, and our customers that the dietary supplement industry is committed to manufacturing and marketing high quality, safe and beneficial products that have a valuable and appropriate role in a wellness regimen. This industry is likewise committed to ensuring that consumers receive truthful, accurate and non-misleading information on dietary supplements.

This testimony is submitted on behalf of the five trade associations who collectively represent all segments of the dietary supplement supply chain: ingredient growers, suppliers and processors, manufacturers and retailers. They are: the American Herbal Products Association (AHPA); the Consumer Healthcare Products Association (CHPA); the Council for Responsible Nutrition (CRN); the Natural Products Association (NPA); and the United Natural Products Alliance (UNPA).

Chapter 6- Modern FDA oversight of dietary supplements began with the 1994 enactment of the Dietary Supplement Health and Education Act (DSHEA).[1] This regulatory system now includes the following key elements.

1. Prior to its marketing, the manufacturer of a dietary supplement is responsible for ensuring that the supplement is safe;
2. Manufacturers are only permitted to make certain types of claims, and may not make false or misleading claims of any kind;
3. Manufacturers must abide by current Good Manufacturing Practices (cGMPs);
4. Manufacturers must submit to FDA all reports that they receive of serious adverse events associated with a product that it manufactures; and
5. A manufacturer must submit a notification to FDA before it markets a dietary supplement containing a "New Dietary Ingredient."

Chapter 7- Dietary supplements are substances you might use to add nutrients to your diet or to lower your risk of health problems, like osteoporosis or arthritis. Dietary supplements come in the form of pills, capsules, powders, gel tabs, extracts, or liquids. They might contain vitamins, minerals, fiber, amino acids, herbs or other plants, or enzymes. Sometimes, the ingredients in dietary supplements are added to foods, including drinks. A doctor's prescription is not needed to buy dietary supplements.

Chapter 8- People use dietary supplements for a wide assortment of reasons. Some seek to compensate for diets, medical conditions, or eating habits that limit the intake of essential vitamins and nutrients. Other people look to them to boost energy or to get a good night's sleep. Postmenopausal women consider using them to counter a sudden drop in estrogen levels.

Chapter 9- Many people take dietary supplements in an effort to be well and stay healthy. With so many dietary supplements available and so many claims made about their health benefits, how can a consumer decide what's safe and effective? This fact sheet provides a general overview of dietary supplements, discusses safety considerations, and suggests sources for additional information.

In: Dietary Supplements: What Seniors Need to… ISBN: 978-1-61761-285-5
Editors: Thomas H. Felton

Chapter 1

OPENING STATEMENT OF SENATOR HERB KOHL, SENATE SPECIAL COMMITTEE ON AGING, HEARING – "DIETARY SUPPLEMENTS: WHAT SENIORS NEED TO KNOW"

Good afternoon. I'd like to thank our witnesses for participating in today's hearing on dietary supplements. The use of dietary supplements, which can take the form of vitamins, minerals, fiber, or other nutritional products, has grown substantially over the past few decades. Recent surveys indicate that at least 40 percent of American adults consume these products, many of which can serve as a valuable and nutritional addition to daily diets. Today we will address concerns that have arisen over whether the marketing and manufacturing of these products meet the standards that American consumers deserve.

Dietary supplements have become a multi-billion dollar industry. In 2006, Americans reportedly spent $23 billion on herbal and specialty supplements, which is almost half the amount they spent on prescription drugs. However, several consumer safety issues arise with these products. Because dietary supplements are available overthe-counter, consumers sometimes take them in addition to, or even as a replacement for, other prescription medication or drugs without consulting their doctors or receiving notification of potentially harmful interactions.

In fact, accurate information is not always easily accessible to the average consumer. The number of scientific studies conducted on the safety or efficacy of herbal supplements is limited, and, unlike pharmaceutical drugs, these supplements are not subject to FDA approval before being marketed and sold. In addition, claims made about these products in advertisements are subject to only limited regulation.

In 2007, the FDA released Good Manufacturing Practices, or GMPs, that began to address some these problems. Though it took thirteen years to complete them, these guidelines are intended to improve the safety and production of dietary supplements. The industry itself has stepped up oversight efforts, and has taken an active role in monitoring its own practices and helping both the FDA and the Federal Trade Commission identify and effectively deal with misleading ads and unfair marketing.

Despite these positive developments, we'll hear today that legitimate concerns remain about the industry. A Government Accountability Office investigation uncovered both improper advertising and marketing of dietary supplements, as well as the existence of contaminants such as mercury, lead, and pesticides in certain products. While the levels of contaminants have not set off alarms with federal regulatory officials or scientists, some exceed allowable limits. As part of their investigation, GAO referred marketing and contaminant samples to FDA and FTC for further review and possible action.

Given these findings, it is obvious that more must be done. I look forward to working with my colleagues in the Senate, including Senators Harkin and Hatch, and Senators McCain and Dorgan, who have long taken an interest in dietary supplement issues, to ensure that meaningful provisions addressing these issues are included in the Food Safety Act. We need to be sure companies are properly registered, including their product lists, so that FDA has the ability to identify and act on safety concerns. Since two-thirds of consumers believe the government requires supplement labels to contain warnings about potential side effects or dangers, we must ensure consumers receive comprehensive information about the safety of these products by requiring warning labels on products that contain ingredients known to have adverse effects or harmful interactions with prescription drugs.

We should encourage vigorous oversight to reduce and eliminate dangerous contaminants, even in small amounts. We need to ensure that FDA has the authority to recall products that are found to harm those who take them. And finally, as FDA authority expands, we need to continue to provide them with the resources to do these things. Last year I was successful in securing a $152 million increase for FDA's food safety oversight, and I will continue to advocate for additional funding in the future.

Now, let's be clear that no one is suggesting that consumers should not be able to take vitamins or other dietary supplements. Our concern is that they be able to do so safely. American consumers should have access to comprehensive, accurate information about these products, so they are empowered to make the best decisions about their own health.

Thank you once again to today's witnesses.

In: Dietary Supplements: What Seniors Need to... ISBN: 978-1-61761-285-5
Editors: Thomas H. Felton

Chapter 2

HERBAL DIETARY SUPPLEMENTS: EXAMPLES OF DECEPTIVE OR QUESTIONABLE MARKETING PRACTICES AND POTENTIALLY DANGEROUS ADVICE

United States Government Accountability Office

WHY GAO DID THIS STUDY

Recent studies have shown that use of herbal dietary supplements—chamomile, echinacea, garlic, ginkgo biloba, and ginseng—by the elderly within the United States has increased substantially. Sellers, such as retail stores, Web sites, and distributors, often claim these supplements help improve memory, circulation, and other bodily functions. GAO was asked to determine (1) whether sellers of herbal dietary supplements are using deceptive or questionable marketing practices and (2) whether selected herbal dietary supplements are contaminated with harmful substances.

To conduct this investigation, GAO investigated a nonrepresentative selection of 22 storefront and mail-order retailers of herbal dietary supplements. Posing as elderly consumers, GAO investigators asked sales staff (by phone and in person) at each retailer a series of questions regarding herbal dietary supplements. GAO also reviewed written marketing language used on approximately 30 retail Web sites. Claims were evaluated against recognized scientific research published by the National Institutes of Health (NIH) and the Food and Drug Administration (FDA). GAO also had an accredited lab test 40 unique popular single-ingredient herbal dietary supplements for the presence of lead, arsenic, mercury, cadmium, organichlorine pesticides, and organophosphorous pesticides.

What GAO Found

Certain dietary supplements commonly used by the elderly were deceptively or questionably marketed. FDA statutes and regulations do not permit sellers to make claims that their products can treat, prevent, or cure specific diseases. However, in several cases, written sales materials for products sold through online retailers claimed that herbal dietary supplements could treat, prevent, or cure conditions such as diabetes, cancer, or cardiovascular disease. When GAO shared these claims with FDA and the Federal Trade Commission (FTC), both agreed that the claims were improper and likely in violation of statutes and regulations. In addition, while posing as elderly customers, GAO investigators were often told by sales staff that a given supplement would prevent or cure conditions such as high cholesterol or Alzheimer's disease. To hear clips of undercover calls, see http://www.gao.gov/products/GAO-10-662T. Perhaps more dangerously, GAO investigators were given potentially harmful medical advice. For example, a seller stated it was not a problem to take ginkgo biloba with aspirin to improve memory; however, FDA warns that combining aspirin and ginkgo biloba can increase a person's risk of bleeding. In another case, a seller stated that an herbal dietary supplement could be taken instead of a medication prescribed by a doctor. GAO referred these sellers to FDA and FTC for appropriate action. The table below includes several deceptive claims made by sellers.

GAO also found trace amounts of at least one potentially hazardous contaminant in 37 of the 40 herbal dietary supplement products tested, though none in amounts considered to pose an acute toxicity hazard. All 37 supplements tested positive for trace amounts of lead; of those, 32 also contained mercury, 28 cadmium, 21 arsenic, and 18 residues from at least one pesticide. The levels of heavy metals found do not exceed any FDA or Environmental Protection Agency (EPA) regulations governing dietary supplements or their raw ingredients, and FDA and EPA officials did not express concern regarding any immediate negative health consequences from consuming these 40 supplements. While the manufacturers GAO spoke with were concerned about finding any contaminants in their supplements, they noted that the levels identified were too low to raise any issues internal product testing.

Mr. Chairman and Members of the Committee:

Thank you for the opportunity to discuss findings from our investigation into the manufacture and marketing of selected herbal dietary supplements commonly used by the elderly.[1] The Dietary Supplement Health and Education Act of 1994 (DSHEA) defines dietary supplements as products that, among other things, are intended for ingestion to supplement the diet, labeled as dietary supplements, and not represented as conventional foods or as a sole items of a meal or diet.[2] Recent studies have shown that use of herbal dietary supplements, such as chamomile, echinacea, garlic, ginkgo biloba, and ginseng, by the elderly in the United States has increased substantially.[3]

Deceptive Marketing Claims for Herbal Supplements Found by GAO Investigators

Claim	Comments
Garlic prevents obesity and diabetes and cures cardiovascular disease.	NIH does not recognize this herbal supplement as a treatment for obesity, diabetes, or cardiovascular disease.
Ginseng cures diseases, including cancer.	NIH specifically recommends that breast and uterine cancer patients avoid this product, as it may have an adverse interaction with some cancer drugs.
Garlic can be taken in lieu of prescribed high blood pressure medication.	Evidence that this product reduces high blood pressure is unclear, and both NIH and FDA state that no dietary supplement can take the place of prescribed medicines.
Ginkgo biloba can be taken with a daily aspirin prescription.	Taking this product with aspirin may increase the risk of bleeding.
Ginkgo biloba treats Alzheimer's disease, depression, and impotence.	No clear scientific evidence supports any of these treatment claims.

Source: GAO.

In 2000, we reported that consumers did not consistently receive clear, scientifically supported information concerning products' health benefits so they could make informed dietary choices. Further, we have reported that consumers faced health risks because federal laws and agencies' efforts did not effectively and consistently ensure that dietary supplements were safe.[4] Most recently, we expressed concern that weaknesses in the regulatory system may increase the likelihood of unsafe products reaching the market, and a lack of consumer knowledge increases the potential health risks associated with uninformed consumption.[5] At your request, we determined (1) whether sellers of herbal dietary supplements are using deceptive or questionable marketing practices to encourage the use of these products and (2) whether selected herbal dietary supplements are contaminated with harmful substances.

To determine whether sellers of herbal dietary supplements are using deceptive or questionable marketing practices to encourage the use of these products, we investigated a nonrepresentative selection of 22 storefront and mail-order retailers. We identified these retailers by searching online using search terms likely to be used by actual consumers and by observing newspaper advertisements. Posing as elderly potential consumers, we asked sales staff at each retailer a series of questions regarding the potential health benefits of herbal dietary supplements as well as potential interactions with other common over-the-counter and prescription drugs. We also reviewed written marketing language used on approximately 30 retail Web sites.[6] We evaluated the accuracy of product marketing claims against health benefit evaluations published through the National Institutes of Health (NIH) and Food and Drug Administration (FDA). While our work focused on herbal dietary supplements, we also evaluated claims made regarding nonherbal supplement products recommended to us during undercover storefront visits and telephone calls.

To determine whether selected herbal dietary supplements are contaminated with harmful substances, we purchased 40 unique single-ingredient herbal supplement products from 40 different manufacturers and submitted them to an accredited laboratory for analysis. We selected the types of herbs to purchase based on recent surveys about the supplements usage of the elderly. These surveys identified the most commonly used herbs among the elderly as chamomile, echinacea, garlic, ginkgo biloba, ginseng, peppermint, saw palmetto, and St. John's wort. We purchased these 40 unique products from a combination of retail chain storefronts and online or mail-order retailers; these retailers were selected independently from those selected for evaluation of marketing practices. For each online retailer, we selected brands based primarily on relative popularity according to the site's list of top sellers. One unopened, manufacturer-sealed bottle of each of these 40 products was submitted to an accredited laboratory where they were screened for the presence of common hazardous contaminants: lead, arsenic, mercury, cadmium, and residues from organichlorine and organophosphorous pesticides. These contaminants were selected based on prevalence and the likelihood of negative health consequences as a result of consumption. We did not independently validate the results received with another lab, or through any other mechanism. The likely negative health consequences from consumption of these contaminants were determined based on a review of relevant health standards and discussions with FDA and Environmental Protection Agency (EPA) experts. For a complete discussion of our scope and methodology, see appendix I. See appendix II for the complete list of contaminants we reviewed.

Our investigative work, conducted from September 2009 through March 2010, was performed in accordance with standards prescribed by the Council of the Inspectors General on Integrity and Efficiency.

BACKGROUND

Herbal dietary supplements are traditionally used to alleviate certain medical conditions, such as anxiety, digestive problems, and depression, and to improve general quality of life. However, for many traditional uses, there is not clear scientific evidence to show that they prevent or treat underlying diseases or conditions. Further, some herbal dietary supplements may interact in a potentially harmful manner with some prescription drugs. For example, according to NIH, St. John's wort can negatively affect the efficacy of antidepressants, HIV treatments, cancer drugs, and anticoagulants, though this is not always noted on product labels. The possibility of adverse drug interactions is one of the reasons that FDA recommends that consumers check with their health practitioners before beginning any supplement regimen. The elderly are particularly at risk from these interactions since recent studies have found that approximately 85 percent of the elderly take at least one prescription drug over the course of a year and 58 percent take three or more. Many herbal supplements have not been exhaustively tested for hazardous interactions with prescription drugs, other supplements, or foods.[7]

Under DSHEA, dietary supplements are broadly presumed safe, and FDA does not have the authority to require them to be approved for safety and efficacy before they enter the market, as it does for drugs. However, a dietary supplement manufacturer or distributor of a supplement with a "new dietary ingredient"—an ingredient that was not marketed in the United States before October 15, 1994—may be required to notify FDA at least 75 days before marketing the product, depending on the history of use of the ingredient.[8] Also, all domestic and foreign companies that manufacture, package, label, or hold dietary supplements must follow FDA's current good manufacturing practice regulations, which outline procedures for ensuring the quality of supplements intended for sale.[9]

Marketing Claims

Under DSHEA, a firm, not FDA, is responsible for determining that any representation or claims made about the dietary supplements it manufactures or distributes are substantiated by adequate evidence to show that they are not false or misleading. Except in the case of a new dietary ingredient, where premarket review for safety data and other information is required by law, a firm does not have to provide FDA with the evidence it relies on to substantiate effectiveness before or after it markets its products. For the most part, FDA relies on postmarket surveillance efforts—such as monitoring adverse event reports it receives from companies, health care practitioners, and individuals; reviewing consumer complaints; and conducting facility inspections—to identify potential safety concerns related to dietary supplements.[10] Once a safety concern is identified, FDA must demonstrate that the dietary supplement presents a significant or unreasonable risk, or is otherwise adulterated, before it can be removed from the market.

A product sold as a dietary supplement cannot suggest on its label or in labeling that it treats, prevents, or cures a specific disease or condition without specific approval from FDA.[11] Under FDA regulations, a manufacturer may submit a health claim petition in order to use a claim on its product labeling that characterizes a relationship between the product and risk of a disease, and FDA may authorize it provided the claims meet certain criteria and are authorized by FDA regulations[12] (e.g., diets high in calcium may reduce the risk of osteoporosis).[13] However, manufacturers may make "qualified health claims" when there is emerging evidence for a relationship between a dietary supplement and reduced risk of a disease or condition, subject to FDA's enforcement discretion. The claim must include specific qualifying language to indicate that the supporting evidence is limited.[14,15]

Dietary supplement labeling may include other claims describing how a dietary ingredient is intended to affect the normal structure or function of the body (e.g. fiber maintains bowel regularity). The manufacturer is responsible for ensuring the accuracy and truthfulness of such claims, but must submit a claim to FDA for review no later than 30 days after marketing it.[16] Because FDA does not confirm the claim—a lack of objection allows the manufacturer to use it—the following disclaimer must be included: "This statement has not been evaluated by the FDA. This product is not intended to diagnose, treat, cure, or prevent any disease." The manufacturer does not need to provide FDA with documentation, and FDA does not test to determine if the claim is true.

In addition, these claims generally may not state that a product is intended to diagnose, mitigate, treat, cure, or prevent a disease or the adverse effects associated with a therapy for a disease, either by naming or describing a specific disease.[17] A claim also cannot suggest an effect on an abnormal condition associated with a natural state or process, such as aging.[18] Context is a consideration; a product's name and labeling cannot imply such an effect by use of pictures or scientific or lay terminology. Finally, a product cannot claim to be a substitute for a product that is a therapy for a disease, or claim to augment a therapy or drug. To make any of these claims, a manufacturer must submit and receive authorization of a health claim petition.

The Federal Trade Commission (FTC) regulates advertising for dietary supplements and other products sold to consumers. FTC receives thousands of consumer complaints each year related to dietary supplements and herbal remedies. FTC has, in the past, taken action against supplement sellers and manufacturers whose advertising was deemed to pose harm to the general public. FDA works with FTC in this area, but FTC's work is directed by different laws.

Harmful Substance Contamination

Consuming high levels of the contaminants for which we tested the 40 products can lead to severe health consequences, such as increased risk of cancer, as noted in table 1. The negative health effects described are, unless otherwise noted, for the acute toxicity in the human body. However, the exact effects of these contaminants on an individual are based on an individual's specific characteristics. For instance, since lead can build up in the human body, the effect of consuming a potentially dangerous level of lead by a 55-year-old man depends on the amount of lead that man has consumed during his lifetime, among other factors.

Table 1. Potential Negative Health Effects of Contaminants Tested for in Selected Herbal Dietary Supplements

Contaminant	Negative health effects
Arsenic	Known to increase risk of lung and skin cancer. Long-term exposure can cause skin pigment changes and a thickening of the skin of the hands and feet.
Cadmium	Known to cause increased risk of leukemia and testicular tumors. Long-term exposure to lower levels can lead to kidney disease, lung damage, and fragile bones.
Lead	May cause increased risk of lung, stomach, and bladder cancer.
Mercury	May cause fever, insomnia, and mood shifts. High levels may cause blindness, deafness, and long-term exposure may cause severe renal damage.
Carbofuran	Cholinesterase inhibitor.[a]
Chlorpyrifos	Light exposure may cause headaches, blurred vision, watery eyes, dizziness, confusion, diarrhea, and change in heart rate. Heavy exposure may cause seizures, coma, and death.
p,p-DDE[b]	May increase risk of liver and thyroid tumors.
gamma-HCH	May cause liver or kidney problems.
HCB	May cause liver, thyroid, and kidney damage; may increase risk of liver, kidney, and thyroid cancer.

Sources: Agency for Toxic Substances and Disease Registry, EPA risk assessments, and National Toxicology Program.

Note: All pesticides sold or distributed in the United States must be registered by EPA, based on scientific studies showing that they can be used without posing unreasonable risks to people or the environment. Because of advances in scientific knowledge, the law requires that pesticides that were first registered before November 1, 1984, be reregistered to ensure that they meet today's more stringent standards. In evaluating pesticides for reregistration, EPA obtains and reviews a complete set of studies from pesticide producers, describing the human health and environmental effects of each pesticide.

[a]A cholinesterase inhibitor behaves similarly to a neurotoxin and may cause abdominal cramps, diarrhea, nausea, and vomiting.

[b]Dichlorodiphenyldichloroethylene (p,p-DDE) is a breakdown product of the pesticide dichlorodiphenyltrichloroethane (DDT).

Table 2. Regulatory Information for Selected Contaminants

Contaminant	Regulatory information
Arsenic	FDA has limited arsenic in bottled drinking water to .010 parts per million (ppm).[a]
Cadmium	FDA has limited cadmium in bottled drinking water to .005 ppm.
Lead	FDA has limited lead in bottled drinking water to .005 ppm.
Mercury	FDA has limited mercury in bottled drinking water to .002 ppm.
Carbofuran	Carbofuran's use is restricted in the United States due to ecological and health risks. FDA has limited carbofuran in bottled drinking water to .04 ppm.
Chlorpyrifos	EPA residue tolerances for chlorpyrifos in food commodities range from .01 to 20.0 ppm.
p,p-DDE	The use of the parent chemical for this breakdown product has been banned in the United States since 1972.
gamma-HCH	EPA National Primary Drinking Water Regulations limit the level of this pesticide in tap water to .0002 ppm. EPA residue tolerances for gamma-HCH in food commodities range from 4.0 to 7.0 ppm.
HCB[b]	EPA National Primary Drinking Water Regulations limit the level of this pesticide in tap water to .001 ppm.

Source: GAO analysis of FDA and EPA regulations.

[a]Parts per million is a measure equivalent to milligrams of contaminant per kilogram of carrier material or milligrams of contaminant per liter of carrier material.

[b]Hexachlorobenzene (HCB) is subject to a voluntary usage ban by U.S. companies. It is not currently used commercially in the United States, though it was previously used to make fireworks, ammunition, and synthetic rubber.

FDA has not issued any regulations addressing safe or unsafe levels of contaminants in dietary supplements, but both FDA and EPA have set certain advisory levels for contaminants in other foods. The human body's absorption of many contaminants is governed by intake method, so advisory levels for other foods (e.g., drinking water) cannot be strictly applied to dietary supplements. In addition, EPA sets limits on how much pesticide residue can remain on food and feed products. These pesticide residue limits are known as tolerances and are enforced by FDA. If no residue tolerance has been set for a particular pesticide, any product containing that pesticide residue is considered adulterated and its sale is prohibited by law. See table 2 for a summary of the regulations issued by FDA or EPA regarding some of the contaminants we tested for.

Table 3. Cases of Deceptive Marketing and Questionable Practices

Case	Product	Deceptive or questionable marketing claim/practice	Comment
1	Ginkgo biloba	Product labeling states it "Effectively treats Alzheimer's Disease, depression, impotence, memory … and more."	Several NIH studies have shown ginkgo to be ineffe-ctive at reducing the risk of Alzheimer's, or otherwise enhancing memory. Other studies have shown that there may be minor allevi-ation of depression in elde-rly patients taking ginkgo, but overall, there is not enough evidence to form a clear conclusion.
2	Garlic	Product labeling states that it prevents and/or cures cardiovascular disease, cancer, obesity, and diabetes.	Only a drug can claim to cure a disease, according to FDA and NIH. As a treatm-ent for these conditions, experts typically recomm-end healthy eating, regular physical activity, and in some cases FDA-approved drugs, not this herbal diet-ary supplement. In addition, no studies suggest that this product can cure or prevent any of these conditions.
3	Ginseng	Product labeling states that it possesses a "Powerful Anti-cancer Function" and can prevent diabetes, among other questionable claims.	NIH states that there is no clear evidence to support that this supplement can prevent cancer or cardiovascular diseases, and more research is needed. While this supplement may lower blood sugar levels in patients with type 2 diabetes, the long-term effects are not clear, and NIH recommends that patients should instead use more proven therapies.
4	Garlic	Product labeling states that "it is extremely helpful in	Some research suggests that this herb may reduce the

Table 3.

Case	Product	Deceptive or questionable marketing claim/practice	Comment
		treating any form of flu or colds, from a mild head cold to pneumonia. [It] is useful for bronchial conditions such as inflammatory disease, asthma, tuberculosis …"	severity of upper respiratory tract infections. However, according to NIH, better studies need to be performed to confirm this effect in humans.
5	Garlic	Product labeling states that "Hundreds of scientific studies have proven [this product] to be number one, working to enhance the body's immune function, protect cells from free radical damage, and reduce cardiovascular risk factors, including issues with blood pressure, cholesterol …"	While this herb may help with certain conditions, enhancement of the body's immune function is not a recognized benefit. Studies have shown that this herb may lower bad cholesterol and blood pressure by a small amount, but the long-term effects are not known. In addition, the effects on good cholesterol are unclear. Further, the seller does not disclose details about the "hundreds of scientific studies" cited in the product labeling.
6	Chamomile	Product labeling states that possible benefits of chamomile include the alleviation of insomnia, diverticular disorder, gum disease, and gingivitis.	Dietary supplements are not a recommended course of treatment for any of these conditions, according to FDA. While chamomile has traditionally been used as a sleep aid, there is a lack of scientific evidence supporting its effectiveness in treating insomnia, according to NIH. For the other conditions, recommended treatments often include lifestyle changes, drugs, and surgery.
7	Enzyme[a]	Publicity materials for this product include a rebuttal of an FDA disclaimer regarding the product's claim to guard against memory issues.	FDA reviewed the supplement and determined that there is little scientific evidence that it reduces the risk of dementia or cognitive dysfunction in the elderly.

Table 3. (Continued)

Case	Product	Deceptive or questionable marketing claim/practice	Comment
8	Garlic	Sales staff informed us that this herbal dietary supplement could be taken in lieu of high blood pressure medicine.	While this herb may lower blood pressure, better studi-es are needed to confirm this benefit, and NIH does not recommend it as a treatment for high blood pressure.
9	Ginkgo biloba	Sales staff informed us that there are no side effects to taking the product with aspirin.	FDA warns that if this pro-duct is taken with certain drugs (including aspirin), it can increase the potential for internal bleeding.
10	Ginkgo biloba	Sales staff informed us that by using this supplement, the use of aspirin is no longer needed.	NIH advises consumers to talk to their health care providers before taking any herbal medicines or supple-ments and before starting or ending any drug regimen.

Source: GAO.

[a]The product described here is not an herbal dietary supplement, but was recommended by sales staff at several retailers to help with memory issues.

Deceptive or Questionable Marketing Claims May Lead to Harm for Elderly Consumers of Herbal Supplements

Our investigation found examples of deceptive or questionable marketing and sales practices for dietary supplements popular among the elderly (see table 3). The most egregious practices included suspect marketing claims that a dietary supplement prevented or cured extremely serious diseases, such as cancer and cardiovascular disease. Other dietary supplements were claimed to mitigate age-related medical conditions, such as Alzheimer's disease and diverticular disorder. We also found some claims that followed FDA's labeling regulations and guidelines, but could still be considered deceptive or questionable and provide consumers with inaccurate information. In addition, while conducting in-person and telephone conversations with dietary supplements sellers, our investigators, posing as elderly consumers, were given potentially harmful medical advice by sales staff, including that they could take supplements in lieu of prescription medication. In making these claims, sellers put the health of consumers at risk. A link to selected audio clips from these calls is available at: http://www.gao.gov/products/GAO-10-662T.

Below are details on several cases in which herbal supplement marketing practices were deceptive or questionable and sometimes posed health risks to consumers. All cases of deceptive or questionable marketing and inappropriate medical advice have been referred to FDA and FTC for appropriate action.

Case 2: In online materials, this garlic supplement included claims that it would (1) prevent and cure cardiovascular disease, (2) prevent and cure tumors and cancer, (3) prevent obesity, and (4) reduce glycemia to prevent diabetes. According to NIH, all these claims are unproven, and garlic is not recommended for treating these conditions. In fact, for several of these conditions, garlic may interact adversely with common FDA-approved drug treatments. Nowhere in this product's marketing materials does the seller suggest that consumers should consult their health care providers prior to taking its supplement. While NIH recognizes that garlic may have some anticancer properties, the agency notes that additional clinical trials are needed to conclude whether these properties are strong enough to prevent or treat cancer. Further, studies have shown that garlic may alter the levels of some cancer drugs in the human body, lessening their effectiveness. For diabetes, there are no studies that confirm that garlic lowers blood sugar or increases the release of insulin in humans. In fact, NIH recommends caution when combining garlic with medications that lower blood sugar, and further suggests that patients taking insulin or oral drugs for diabetes be monitored closely by qualified health care professionals.

Case 3: According to its labeling, this ginseng supplement—which costs $500 for a 90-day supply—cures diseases, effectively prevents diabetes and cardiovascular disease, and prevents cancer or halts its progression. These claims are unproven—no studies confirm that ginseng can prevent or cure any disease. In fact, NIH recommends that breast and uterine cancer patients avoid ginseng. In addition, ginseng may adversely interact with cancer drugs. The product labeling claims do not differentiate between type 1 and type 2 diabetes. According to NIH, ginseng's effect on patients with type 1 diabetes is not well studied. While ginseng may lower blood sugar levels in patients with type 2 diabetes, the long-term effects of such a treatment program are unclear, and it is not known what doses are safe or effective. NIH specifically recommends that consumers with type 2 diabetes use proven therapies instead of this supplement.

Case 7: While our investigators posed as consumers purchasing dietary supplements, sales staff provided them with an informational booklet regarding an enzyme that claims to "[defend] us against dementia and Alzheimer's, exhibiting a truly miraculous capacity to optimize mental performance and fight off cognitive decline." In fact, FDA reviewed the scientific evidence for the active ingredient of this supplement and found that it was not adequate to make such a claim. Because the agency considered such a health claim potentially misleading, FDA provided for the use of a qualified health claim that contains a disclaimer that must accompany the health claim in all labeling in which these claims appear. While the booklet we received does state the FDA disclaimer on the first page, the manufacturer follows it with a rejoinder: "The very cautious language of these claims, which FDA mandates can only be stated word for word, is at best a grudging concession to the extensive clinical research done with [this supplement]. Considering this agency's legendary toughness against dietary supplements, FDA's willingness to go this far with the [disclaimer] suggests that the FDA must be sure it is safe to take and also that the FDA is unable to deny [this supplement] can improve human brain function."

Case 8: One of our fictitious consumers visited a supplement specialty store looking for a product that would help with high blood pressure. The sales representative recommended a garlic supplement and stated that the product could be taken in lieu of prescribed blood pressure medication. According to NIH, while this herb may lower blood pressure by a small amount, the scientific evidence is unclear. NIH does not recommend this supplement as a treatment for high blood pressure and warns patients to use caution while taking this product with other drugs or supplements that can lower blood pressure. Further, it is not recommended that a consumer start or stop a course of treatment without consulting with his or her health care provider. Even if a sales representative is licensed to dispense medical advice, he or she still does not know the consumer's patient history, including other drug programs, allergies, and medical conditions, making it potentially dangerous for the sales representative to provide medical advice.

Case 9: At a supplement specialty store, one of our investigators posed as an elderly consumer who was having difficulty remembering things. A sales representative recommended one of the store's ginkgo biloba supplements. The consumer told the representative that he takes aspirin everyday and asked if it was safe to take aspirin and ginkgo biloba together. The sales representative told him that it is completely safe to take the two together. However, according to FDA, if aspirin is taken with the recommended product, it can increase the potential for internal bleeding.

We spoke to FDA and FTC regarding these 10 claims, and they agreed that the statements made in product labeling for cases 1 through 6 are largely improper, as the labeling suggests that each product has an effect on a specific disease. For case 7, FDA stated that while the specific claims discussed here are allowable, depending on the context in which they were made, FDA might consider the totality of marketing materials to be improper. FDA also agreed that the claims made to our undercover investigators in cases 8 and 10 were questionable or likely constituted improper disease claims, but that to take action, additional information as to the prevalence and context of the claims would be necessary. For case 9, FDA noted that, since the statement made by sales staff was safe usage information, not a claim about the product's effects, it would not violate FDA regulations, unless the agency could develop other evidence to show that the claim was false or misleading or constituted an implied disease claim. In addition, FDA and NIH both noted that by definition, no dietary supplement can treat, prevent, or cure any disease.

TRACE CONTAMINANTS FOUND IN SELECTED HERBAL DIETARY SUPPLEMENTS, BUT NONE POSE AN ACUTE TOXICITY HAZARD TO HUMANS

We found trace amounts of at least one potentially hazardous contaminant in 37 of the 40 herbal dietary supplement products we tested, though none of the contaminants were found in amounts considered to pose an acute toxicity hazard to humans.[19] Specifically, all 37 supplements tested positive for trace amounts of lead. Thirty-two also contained mercury, 28 contained cadmium, 21 contained arsenic, and 18 contained residues from at least one pesticide.[20] See appendixes III and IV for the complete results of these tests.

The levels of contaminants found do not exceed any FDA or EPA regulations governing dietary supplements or their raw ingredients, and FDA and EPA officials did not express concern regarding any immediate negative health consequences from consuming these 40 supplements. However, because

EPA has not set pesticide tolerance limits for the main ingredients of the herbal dietary supplements we tested, the pesticide contaminants exceed FDA advisory levels. FDA agreed that 16 of the 40 supplements we tested would be considered in violation of U.S. pesticide tolerances if FDA, using prescribed testing procedures, confirmed our results. We note that 4 of the residues detected are from pesticides that currently have no registered use in the United States.[21] According to FDA, scientific research has not been done on the long-term health effects from consumption of such low levels of many of these specific contaminants, as current technology cannot detect these trace contaminants when they are diluted in human bloodstreams. We have referred these products to FDA for its review.

After reviewing test results with EPA and FDA officials, we also spoke with several of the manufacturers of supplements that had trace amounts of contaminants.[22] The manufacturers we spoke with stated that they ensure that their products are tested for contamination, and that these tests have shown that their products do not contain contaminants in excess of regulatory standards. Manufacturers also stated that they comply with all FDA regulations and follow good manufacturing practices as defined by the agency. While the manufacturers we spoke with were concerned about finding any contaminants in their supplements, they noted that the levels identified were too low to raise any issues during their own internal product testing processes.

Mr. Chairman, this concludes my statement. I would be pleased to answer any questions that you or other members of the committee may have at this time.

APPENDIX I. SCOPE AND METHODOLOGY

To determine whether sellers of herbal dietary supplements are using deceptive or questionable marketing practices to encourage the use of these products, we investigated a nonrepresentative selection of 22 storefront and mail-order retailers selling herbal dietary supplements. We identified these retailers by searching online using search terms likely to be used by actual consumers and by observing newspaper advertisements. Posing as elderly customers, we asked sales staff at each company a series of questions regarding the potential health benefits of herbal dietary supplements as well as potential interactions with other common over-the-counter and prescription drugs.[23] While our work focused on herbal dietary supplements, we also evaluated claims made regarding nonherbal supplement products during undercover storefront visits and telephone calls. We also reviewed written marketing language used on approximately 30 retail Web sites. We evaluated the accuracy of product marketing claims against health benefit evaluations published through the National Institutes of Health and Food and Drug Administration (FDA).

To determine whether selected herbal dietary supplements were contaminated with harmful substances, we purchased 40 unique single-ingredient herbal supplement products from 40 different manufacturers and submitted them to an accredited laboratory for analysis. We selected the types of herbs to purchase based on recent surveys about the supplements usage of the elderly, defined for this chapter as individuals over the age of 65. These surveys identified the most commonly used herbs among the elderly as chamomile, echinacea, garlic, ginkgo biloba, ginseng, peppermint, saw palmetto, and St. John's wort.

We purchased these 40 unique products from a combination of retail chain storefronts and online or mail-order retailers. For each online retailer, we selected products based primarily on relative popularity according to the site's list of top sellers. At each retail chain storefront, because of limited selection, we selected only items that would be expected to be sold at all chain locations. All 40 products were submitted to an accredited laboratory where they were screened for the presence of lead, arsenic, mercury, cadmium, and residues from organichlorine and organophosphorous pesticides. These contaminants were selected based on prevalence and the likelihood of negative health consequences due to consumption. The recommended daily intake levels of these contaminants and the likely negative health consequences because of consumption were determined based on a review of relevant health standards and discussions with FDA and Environmental Protection Agency experts.

For each herbal dietary supplement product, we submitted one unopened, manufacturer-sealed bottle to the laboratory for analysis. To identify levels of arsenic, cadmium, lead, and mercury, products were analyzed using inductively coupled plasma mass spectrometry according to method AOAC 993.14. Detection limits for these contaminants were .075 milligrams/kilogram, .010 milligrams/kilogram, .005 milligrams/kilogram, and .050 nanograms/gram, respectively. To identify levels of pesticide residues, products were analyzed using a variety of residue-specific methods, including those methods published in the FDA *Pesticide Analytical Manual*. We did not independently validate the results received with another lab or through any other mechanism. See appendix II for a complete list of analytes and their related detection levels.

Appendix II. Full List of Analytes and Detection Limits

Analyte	Detection limit (ppm)[a]	Analyte	Detection limit (ppm)[a]
(2-Ethylhexyl)-Diphenylphosphate	0.01	cis-Chlordane	0.01
Acrinathrin	0.01	Clomazone	0.01
Aldrin	0.01	Coumaphos	0.01
Allethrin	0.01	Cyanazine	0.01
alpha-BHC	0.01	Cyanophos	0.01
Ametryn	0.01	Cycloate/Ro Neet	0.01
Aminocarb	0.01	Cycluron	0.01
Amitraz	0.05	Cyhalothrin lambda	0.01
Aniten/Flurecol Butyl Ester	0.05	Cymiazole	0.01
Arsenic	0.075	Cypermethrin	0.02
Atrazine	0.01	Cyproconazole	0.01
Azinphos-methyl	0.01	Cyprodinil	0.01
Azoxystrobin	0.01	Dacthal (DCPA)	0.01
Benalaxyl	0.01	DEF	0.02
Bendiocarb	0.01	delta-BHC	0.01
Benfluralin	0.01	Deltamethrin	0.01
beta-BHC	0.01	Desmedipham	0.01
Bifenthrin	0.01	Desmetryn	0.01
Biphenyl	0.02	Di-allate	0.01
Bromopropylate	0.01	Diazinon	0.01
Bufencarb	0.01	Diazinon (O Analog)	0.01
Bupirimate	0.01	Dichlobenil	0.05
Buprofezin	0.01	Dicloran	0.02
Butylate	0.01	Dieldrin	0.01
Cadmium	0.01	Diethofencarb	0.01
Carbaryl	0.01	Difenoconazole	0.01
Carbofuran	0.01	Dimethachlor	0.01
Carbofuran 3-OH	0.01	Dimethoate	0.01

Carbosulfan	0.02	Diniconazole	0.01
Carboxin	0.01	Dioxacarb	0.01
Chlordene, beta	0.02	Dioxathion	0.05
Chlordene, gamma	0.02	Diphenamid	0.01
Chlordimeform (CDF)	0.01	Disulfoton	0.01
Chlorfenvinphos (Total Isomers E, Z)	0.01	d-Phenothrin	0.01
Chlorobenzilate	0.01	Edifenphos	0.01
Chloroneb	0.01	Endosulfan I (alpha-endosulfan)	0.01
Chloropropylate	0.01	Endosulfan II (beta-Endosulfan)	0.01
Chlorothalonil	0.01	Endosulfan sulphate	0.01
Chlorpyrifos (Dursban)	0.01	Endrin	0.01
Chlorpyrifos-methyl	0.01	EPN	0.01
Chlorpyrifos-O-analogue	0.01	Epoxiconazole	0.01
EPTC/Eptam	0.01	Isocarbamid	0.01
Esfenvalerate-2	0.01	Isofenphos	0.01
Etaconazole	0.01	Isoprocarb	0.01
Ethafluralin	0.03	Isopropalin	0.01
Ethiofencarb	0.01	Isoprothiolane	0.01
Ethiolate	0.01	Isoproturon	0.01
Ethion	0.01	Kresoxim-methyl	0.01
Ethofumesate	0.01	Lead	0.005
Ethoprop (Ethoprophos)	0.01	Lenacil	0.01
Ethoxyquin	0.01	Linuron	0.01
Etobenzanid	0.01	Malathion	0.01
Etofenprox	0.01	Malathion OA (Malaoxon)	0.01
Etridiazole	0.01	Mercury	0.05[b]
Fenamiphos	0.01	Metalaxyl	0.01
Fenarimol	0.01	Methidathion	0.01
Fenazaquin	0.01	Methiocarb	0.01
Fenbuconazole	0.01	Methoprotryne	0.01
Fenchlorphos	0.01	Methoxychlor, o,o'	0.01
Fenitrothion	0.02	Methoxychlor, p,p'	0.01
Fenobucarb	0.01	Methyl Parathion	0.02

Appendix II (Continued)			
Fenoxycarb	0.01	Metolachlor	0.01
Fenpropimorph	0.01	Metolcarb	0.01
Fenthion	0.01	Metribuzin	0.01
Fenvalerate	0.01	Mevinphos	0.01
flopet	0.01	Mexacarbate	0.01
Fluchloralin	0.04	MGK-264	0.01
Flucythrinate (Total Isomers)	0.01	Mirex	0.01
Fludioxonil	0.01	Molinate	0.01
Flusilazole	0.01	Monocrotophos	0.01
Flutolanil	0.01	Monolinuron	0.01
Fluvalinate	0.02	Myclobutanil	0.01
Fonofos	0.01	Naphthalene Acetamide	0.01
Gamma-cyhalothrin	0.01	Napropamide	0.01
gamma-HCH (Lindane)	0.01	Nitralin	0.01
Heptachlor	0.01	Nitrofen	0.01
Heptachlor Epoxide (cis, trans)	0.01	Nitrothal-isopropyl	0.02
Heptenophos	0.01	nonachlor cis-	0.01
Hexachlorobenzene (HCB)	0.01	Nonachlor trans-	0.01
Hexaconazole	0.01	Norea	0.02
Hexazinone	0.01	Nuarimol	0.01
Iprodione	0.02	o,p-DDE	0.01
o,p-DDT	0.01	Quintozene (PCNB)	0.02
Oxydemeton Methyl Sulfone	0.05	Resmethrin	0.01
p,p-DDE	0.01	S 421 (Octachlordipropylether)	0.02
p,p-DDT	0.01	Sethoxydim	0.02
Parathion-ethyl	0.01	Simazine	0.01
Penconazole	0.01	Simetryn	0.01
Pendimethalin	0.01	Sulfotep	0.01
Pentachloroaniline	0.01	Sulprofos	0.01
Pentachlorobenzene	0.01	Tebuconazole	0.01
Pentachlorobenzonitrile	0.01	Tebufenpyrad	0.01
Pentachlorothioanisole	0.01	Tebutam	0.01

Permethrin-cis	0.01	Tebuthiuron	0.01
Permethrin-trans	0.01	Tecnazene	0.01
Phenmedipham	0.01	Terbufos	0.01
Phorate	0.01	Terbumeton	0.01
Phorate-sulfone	0.02	Terbuthylazine	0.01
Phorate-sulfoxide	0.01	Terbutryn	0.01
Phosalone	0.01	Tetrachloroaniline, 2,3,4,6-	0.01
Phosmet	0.01	Tetrachlorvinphos	0.01
Pirimicarb	0.01	Tetraconazole	0.01
Pirimifos-methyl	0.01	Tetradifon	0.01
Prochloraz	0.01	Tetramethrin	0.01
Procymidon	0.01	Thiabendazole	0.01
Profenofos	0.01	Tolclofos-methyl	0.01
Profluralin	0.01	Tolylfluanid	0.01
Promecarb	0.01	Tralkoxydim	0.05
Prometon	0.01	trans-Chlordane	0.01
Prometryn	0.01	Triadimefon	0.01
Propachlor	0.01	Triadimenol	0.01
Propanil	0.01	Triallate	0.01
Propargite	0.01	Triazophos	0.01
Propham	0.01	Tricyclazol	0.01
Propiconazole	0.01	Trifloxystrobin	0.01
Prothiofos	0.01	Triflumizole	0.01
Pyracarbolid	0.01	Trifluralin	0.01
Pyrazophos	0.01	Trimethacarb 2.3.5-	0.01
Pyridaphenthion	0.01	Trimethacarb 3.4.5-	0.01
Pyrimethanil	0.01	Triticonazole	0.01
Pyriproxyfen	0.01	Vinclozolin	0.02
Quinalphos	0.01		
Quinoxyfen	0.01		

Source: GAO, based on laboratory methodology.

[a] Parts per million is a measure equivalent to milligrams per kilogram or milligrams per liter.

[b] Mercury results appear as parts per billion.

APPENDIX III. CONTAMINANTS FOUND IN SELECTED HERBAL DIETARY SUPPLEMENTS (IN PARTS PER MILLION)

Sample	Herb	Arsenic[a,b]	Cadmium[a,b]	Lead[a,b]	Mercury[b,c]	Number of pesticides[d]
1	Saw palmetto	nd	0.011	0.024	1.210	0
2	Echinacea	0.090	0.348	0.106	1.170	0
3	Echinacea	0.093	0.030	0.043	nd	0
4	Echinacea	0.226	0.069	1.290	6.960	1
5	St. John's wort	0.391	0.090	0.353	0.980	2
6	St. John's wort	0.153	0.033	0.587	2.330	0
7	Ginkgo biloba	nd	nd	0.564	1.340	1
8	Garlic	nd	nd	0.046	0.810	1
9	Ginkgo biloba	0.151	nd	0.036	1.480	2
10	Ginkgo biloba	0.162	0.017	0.037	3.420	1
11	Garlic	nd	0.026	0.026	0.620	2
12	Ginseng	0.123	0.057	0.126	10.700	5
13	Peppermint	nd	nd	0.007	2.170	1
14	Saw palmetto	nd	nd	0.011	nd	0
15	Echinacea	0.116	0.016	0.109	4.110	0
16	Ginkgo biloba	0.222	0.030	0.112	6.090	0
17	Garlic	nd	0.040	0.029	1.090	0
18	Saw palmetto	nd	nd	0.026	nd	0
19	St. John's wort	nd	0.011	0.026	0.860	3

Table.

Sample	Herb	Arsenic[a,b]	Cadmium[a,b]	Lead[a,b]	Mercury[b,c]	Number of pesticides[d]
20	Ginseng	0.078	0.127	0.439	1.510	0
21	Garlic	nd	0.062	0.030	0.640	0
22	Chamomile	nd	0.375	0.049	2.900	0
23	Chamomile	0.094	0.146	0.375	2.420	4
24	Peppermint	nd	nd	nd	nd	0
25	Chamomile	nd	nd	nd	nd	0
26	Chamomile	nd	nd	nd	nd	0
27	St. John's wort	0.155	0.054	0.111	0.530	0
28	Garlic	nd	0.050	0.305	0.780	0
29	St. John's wort	0.180	0.062	0.148	0.760	2
30	Peppermint	nd	nd	0.023	nd	1
31	Chamomile	0.286	0.058	0.802	4.260	0
32	Ginkgo biloba	0.524	0.054	0.487	77.800	2
33	Ginseng	0.229	0.105	1.290	32.900	6
34	Ginseng	0.172	nd	0.032	2.110	2
35	Ginseng	0.154	0.156	0.408	5.990	3
36	Saw palmetto	nd	nd	0.008	1.100	0
37	Saw palmetto	nd	0.012	0.125	1.710	0
38	St. John's wort	nd	1.150	0.138	3.000	0
39	Echinacea	0.152	0.032	0.649	6.930	0
40	Ginkgo biloba	0.115	0.025	0.061	nd	2

Source: GAO, based on laboratory analysis.

[a]Parts per million is a measure equivalent to milligrams per kilogram or milligrams per liter.

[b]Results marked as "nd" indicate that the contaminant was not detected in excess of the underlying tests' detection limit (.075 mg/kg for arsenic, .010 mg/kg for cadmium, .005 mg/kg for lead, and .050 ng/g for mercury). A result of "nd" does not mean

that a contaminant does not exist in a sample. It means that if a contaminant is in the product, it appears at a level below the detection limit for that particular test method.

[c]Mercury results appear as parts per billion, a measure equivalent to nanograms per gram or nanograms per milliliter.

[d]For additional details on pesticide residues found, see appendix IV.

APPENDIX IV. PESTICIDE RESIDUES IDENTIFIED IN SELECTED HERBAL DIETARY SUPPLEMENTS (IN PARTS PER MILLION)

Sample no.	Herb	Pesticide residue	Detected level
4[a]	Echinacea	Chlorpyrifos (Dursban)	0.01
5[a]	St. John's wort	Amitraz	0.05
		Propargite	0.04
7[a]	Ginkgo biloba	Phorate-sulfoxide	0.06
8[a]	Garlic	Triadimenol	0.03
9[a]	Ginkgo biloba	Phorate-sulfoxide	0.10
		Triadimenol	0.26
10[a]	Ginkgo biloba	Phorate-sulfoxide	0.06
11[a]	Garlic	Carbofuran	0.04
		gamma-HCH (Lindane)	0.08
12[a]	Ginseng	Azoxystrobin[b]	0.02
		Difenoconazole	0.02
		Flutolanil	0.03
		Tebuconazole	0.02
		Tolclofos-methyl	0.05
13	Peppermint	Propargite[b]	0.16
19[a]	St. John's wort	Azoxystrobin	0.01
		Chlorpyrifos (Dursban)	0.01
		Hexazinone	0.06
23[a]	Chamomile	Flusilazole	0.01
		Metolachlor	0.02
		Tebuconazole	0.04
		Trifloxystrobin	0.01
29[a]	St. John's wort	Amitraz	0.06
		Triadimefon	0.02

Sample no.	Herb	Pesticide residue	Detected level
30	Peppermint	Propargite[b]	0.62
32[a]	Ginkgo biloba	Phorate-sulfoxide	0.01
		Triadimenol	0.06
33[a]	Ginseng	Hexachlorobenzene (HCB)	0.02
		Metalaxyl[b]	0.01
		p,p-DDE	0.02
		Pentachloroaniline	0.28
		Pentachlorothioanisole	0.05
		Pyrimethanil	0.03
34[a]	Ginseng	Metalaxyl[b]	0.03
		Propiconazole	0.02
35[a]	Ginseng	Azoxystrobin[b]	0.03
		Dacthal (DCPA)[b]	0.07
		Pyrimethanil	0.11
40[a]	Ginkgo biloba	Phorate-sulfoxide	0.01
		Triadimenol	0.10

Source: GAO, based on laboratory analysis.

[a]Product would be considered in violation of U.S. pesticide tolerances, should these results be confirmed.

[b]Pesticide residue detected is not considered, by the Food and Drug Administration, to be of regulatory significance.

End Notes

[1] For purposes of this testimony, we defined elderly as people 65 years of age and older.

[2] Pub. L. No. 103-417, § 3, 108 Stat. 4325, 4327 (codified at 21 U.S.C. § 321(ff)).

[3] Herbal supplements are one type of dietary supplement. An herb is a plant or plant part (such as leaves, flowers, or seeds) that is used for its flavor, scent, therapeutic properties, or a combination of these. "Botanical" is often used as a synonym for "herb." An herbal supplement may contain a single herb or mixtures of herbs.

[4] GAO, *Food Safety: Improvements Needed in Overseeing the Safety of Dietary Supplements and "Functional Foods,"* GAO/RCED-00-156 (Washington, D.C.: July 11, 2000).

[5] GAO, *Dietary Supplements: FDA Should Take Further Actions to Improve Oversight and Consumer Understanding*, GAO-09-250 (Washington, D.C.: Jan. 29, 2009).

[6] Our findings are limited to the individual retailers and sales staff we investigated. Our findings cannot be projected to any other retailers or sales representatives.

[7] FDA does not require that herbal supplement manufacturers conduct such testing.

[8] For the products reviewed as part of this testimony, most of the dietary ingredients involved were marketed prior to October 15, 1994, and therefore were not subject to the "new dietary ingredient" approval requirement.

[9] 21 U.S.C. § 342(g) and 21 C.F.R. §§ 111.1 - .610

[10] As of December 22, 2007, dietary supplement companies are required to submit any report received about a serious adverse event to FDA, as mandated by the Dietary Supplement and Nonprescription Drug Consumer Protection Act. (Pub. L. No. 109-462, § 3(a),120 Stat. 3469, 3472 (codified at 21 U.S.C. § 379aa-1)). In addition, companies can voluntarily submit reports about moderate and mild adverse events. Others, such as consumers and health care practitioners, can submit reports of serious, moderate, and mild adverse events on a voluntary basis to FDA.

[11] Labeling refers to the label as well as accompanying material that is used by a manufacturer to promote and market a specific product.

[12] FDA authorizes these types of health claims under the Nutrition Labeling and Education Act of 1990 (Pub. L. No. 101-535, § 3(a), 104 Stat. 2353, 2357-60 (codified at 21 U.S.C. § 321(r))) based on extensive review of the scientific literature, generally as a result of the submission of a health claim petition, using the significant scientific agreement standard to determine that the nutrient/disease relationship is well established.

[13] A manufacturer may, alternately, obtain FDA approval to market its product as a drug intended for the treatment, prevention, cure, mitigation, or diagnosis of a specific disease.

[14] Dietary supplement labeling may contain nutrient content claims, which describe the level of a nutrient or dietary substance in the product using terms such as "free," "high," and "low," or compare the level of a nutrient in a food to that of another food, using terms such as "more," "reduced," and "lite."

[15] The constitutionality of some of FDA's health claim regulations for dietary supplements have been successfully challenged in court. In *Pearson v. Shalala*, 164 F.3d 650 (DC Cir. 1999), the United States Court of Appeals for the District of Columbia Circuit held that while inherently or actually misleading information could be absolutely prohibited, the First Amendment did not permit such a restriction on information that is only potentially misleading. The determination of whether regulation of potentially misleading information is permissible instead requires an analysis of the level of government interest, the potential advancement of the government interest by the regulation, and the reasonableness of the means chosen to accomplish the government's goals.

[16] FDA receives approximately 4,000 such claims submissions per year for one or more claims for one or more products.

[17] FDA defines a disease as "damage to an organ, part, structure, or system of the body such that it does not function properly (e.g., cardiovascular disease), or a state of health leading to such dysfunctioning (e.g., hypertension); except that diseases resulting from essential nutrient deficiencies (e.g., scurvy, pellagra) are not included in this definition."

[18] Some natural states or processes such as aging, menopause, and the menstrual cycle, are not themselves diseases but can be associated with abnormal conditions that are diseases. Two criteria determine if such a condition will be considered a disease: (1) if the condition is uncommon or (2) if the condition can cause significant or permanent harm.

[19] Our results are limited by the tests performed. Since we only tested a single bottle of each sample, our results cannot be projected beyond the single bottle tested. Our results also cannot be projected to any other products from the same manufacturers.

[20] Different forms of mercury have distinctly different adverse effects. The tests we performed to identify mercury levels in supplements do not differentiate between these different forms of mercury.

[21] EPA cancelled all registrations of carbofuran, gamma-HCH (Lindane), and dichlorodiphenyltrichloroethane (DDT), the parent chemical of p,p-DDE. As of December 31, 2009, all related residue tolerances had been revoked. Tolclofos-methyl has never had a U.S. registration, but it is approved for use in other countries.

[22] Discussions with these manufacturers were limited to their manufacturing and quality control processes. We did not question these manufacturers regarding the marketing of their products.

[23] Our findings are limited to the individual retailers and sales staff we investigated. Our findings cannot be projected to any other retailers or sales representatives.

In: Dietary Supplements: What Seniors Need to… ISBN: 978-1-61761-285-5
Editors: Thomas H. Felton

Chapter 3

TESTIMONY OF TOD COOPERMAN, MD., PRESIDENT, CONSUMERLAB.COM TO SENATE SPECIAL COMMITTEE ON AGING, HEARING – "DIETARY SUPPLEMENTS: WHAT SENIORS NEED TO KNOW"

Dear Senator Kohl and Members of the Committee,

I am Dr. Tod Cooperman, the President of ConsumerLab.com, a company that I founded eleven years ago to help consumers identify better quality health and nutrition products based on independent testing. I am accompanied by Dr. William Obermeyer, our Vice President for Research, who spent nine years at the FDA testing food and dietary supplements in the Center for Food Safety and Applied Nutrition.

We appreciate this opportunity to present findings that are particularly relevant to the aging population.

CONSUMERLAB.COM BACKGROUND

ConsumerLab.com's esting is funded by over 40,000 individual and institutional subscribers to ourt website (www.consumerlab.com). We also provide a Voluntary Certification Program and test products for clinical researchers (many funded by the NIH).

Use of Supplements by Seniors

A recent survey of people who receive our free e-newsletter revealed that that *among those aged 65 and older, 32% use 10 or more supplements daily* (Reference 1).

A senior citizen in a vitamin store is a bit like a kid a candy store. However, while the FDA recommends a strict limit on lead contamination in candy, it has not set a limit for supplements. Our tests show that this policy has created a " buyer beware" situation.

General Findings from Supplement Testing

Based on tests of over 2,000 dietary supplements representing over 300 different brands, we find that *one out of four has a quality problem.* Problems have been found in products from every size of manufacturer and are most common in herbal supplements, multivitamins, and products with ingredients that are newer to the market.

The Most Common Problem is a Lack of Ingredient or Substandard Ingredient

Our most recent tests of herbal supplements show that 46% contained less than their expected amounts of key compounds. For example, an "Extra Strength" ginseng an 10% of theproduct claimed amount of expected "ginsenoside" compounds the same product when purchased three years earlier (Reference 2).

Herbal supplements failing to contain claimed or expected amounts of marker compounds (among products selected in recent reviews):

- Echinacea: 5 of 6 failed to contain expected amounts of specific phenolic compounds (Reference 3).
- Garlic: 6 of 14 supplements had too little of the key compound allicin (Reference 4).
- Ginkgo: 4 of 7 supplements failed to contain the expected amounts of individual flavonol compounds, suggesting adulteration to enhance the apparent quality of the ginkgo material (Reference 5).

- Ginseng: 3 out of 13 failed to contain the expected amount of marker ginsenosides (Reference 2).
- Milk thistle: 7 of 10 failed to meet claims of silymarin standardization (Reference 6).
- St. John's wort: 3 of 10 d amounts of hypericin oronly 23% hyperforin (Reference 7).
- Turmeric: 2 of 9 were low in curcuminoids (Reference 8).
- Valerian: 8 of 14 were low in valerenic acids (Reference 9).
- A similar problem exists with certain non-herbal supplements, such as chondroitin (Reference 10).

A major cause of these problems is the reliance by some manufacturers on cheap, non-specific tests which overstate the amount of actual ingredient in raw materials and supplements. More specific tests show the actual amounts to be much lower.

The Next Most Common Problem is Contamination with Lead and Other Heavy Metals

The FDA professes a policy of reducing lead levels to the lowest amount that can be practicably obtained in manufacturing, yet the FDA has neither set nor suggested limits on heavy metals in supplements. The only official limit on lead in supplements is in the State of California. That limit, 0.5 mcg per daily serving typically works out to be slightly higher than the FDA candy limit, but is still very conservative and meaningful. Products sold in California exceeding this limit must carry a warning label (Reference 11). ConsumerLab.com has found that *11% of herbal supplements exceed the California limit for lead.*

Cadmium, a toxin and carcinogen, also occurs in certain herbal supplements, but the FDA has not set a limit on cadmium in supplements. ConsumerLab.com has found 40% of St. John's supplementswort and 14% of valerian supplements to exceed World Health Organization guidelines for cadmium contamination.

Herbal supplements found to exceed California Prop 65 lead limit or the WHO cadmium guidelines:

- Echinacea: 1 of 6 failed for lead (Reference 3).

- Garlic: 2 of 14 failed for lead (Reference 4).
- Ginkgo: 1 of 7 failed for lead (Reference 5).
- Ginseng: 1 out of 13 failed for lead (Reference 2).
- Milk thistle: None of 10 failed for lead (Reference 6).
- St. John's wort: Out of 10 products, 1 failed for lead and 4 failed for cadmium (including thewo product contaminated with lead) (Reference 7).
- Turmeric: 2 of 9 failed for lead (Reference 8).
- Valerian: Out of 14 products, 1 failed for lead and 2 for cadmium (Reference 9).
- The highest levels found by ConsumerLab.com are 16 mcg and 19 mcg of lead, respectively, in daily servings of ginkgo and turmeric supplements (References 5, 8).
- Some chromium supplements are contaminated with a carcinogenic form of chromium, known at hexavalent chromium. The FDA has not established limits for hexavalent chromium in supplements. California has proposed a limit on hexavalent chromium in its water supplies, which equates to 0.12 mcg in a normal daily intake of water. We recently found much higher amounts (1.6 to 26.4 mcg of hexavalent chromium) in three chromium supplements (Reference 12).

While individual products with elevated levels of lead and cadmium are generally not toxic in themselves, they unnecessarily expose Americans to toxins and the effects are cumulative. As noted earlier, many seniors take ten or more supplements daily and additional exposure comes from foods, beverages, and the environment. It would be dangerous to suggest that a single supplement needs to contain a toxic amount of heavy metal to be a threat to health. However, a 2007 report by the FDA on lead contamination in multivitamins made this faulty assumption and has been criticized for doing so (Reference 13).

Unfortunately, the USP may soon adopt an industry proposal permitting 10 micrograms of lead per daily serving of a supplement twenty times higher than the California limit. We think such a lax standard would be a terrible mistake, permitting an individual supplement to exceed the total amount of lead that a child can tolerate (6 mcg), and just a few supplements to surpass the daily threshold for adults (Reference 11).

OTHER PROBLEMS

- Tablets that won't break apart properly to release all of their ingredients (References 5, 10, 14, 15, 16).
- A lack of proper labeling to indicate the parts of the plants used (References 5, 8) and deceptive labeling suggesting more ingredients than actually provided (References 10, 17).
- A lack of voluntary warnings which could help consumers avoid potential problems, such ingredients in excess of known tolerable intake levels (References 18, 19).
- Faulty products left on the market due to inaction by manufacturers or "quiet" announced to retailers but not to the public. (Reference 2)
- Spiking of supplements with prescription drugs, particularly those for erectile dysfunction. (Reference 20)
- Lack of public access to adverse event reports filed by manufacturers with the FDA.

WILL GOOD MANUFACTURING PRACTICES (GMPS) HELP?

Good Manufacturing Practices (GMPs) are now required of most supplement manufacturers to help ensure batch-to-batch uniformity. However, "bad" products , and are, being made u can nder these practices because the GMPs do not include standards for purity and ingredient identity. These standards, and the selection of tests used to measure against them, are left to each manufacturer to determine for itself.

CONCLUSION

Nearly eleven years of product reviews by ConsumerLab.com have shown consistent problems with a significant percentage of dietary supplements, particularly herbal supplements. However, in nearly every supplement category that we test, we do find products that meet high quality standards, showing that this is achievable. If we want our supplements to be the best and safest in the world, we will need better guidance from government establishing rigorous standards and test methods, greater enforcement of current regulations, and more self-regulation from the industry.

In my written testimony, you will find additional statistics, information, and references.

References

[1] ConsumerLab.com Survey of Supplement Users. (2010). Report. February 1, 2010 news release. http://www.consumerlab.com/news/Supplement_Survey_Report/1_31_2010/

[2] ConsumerLab.com Product Review of Ginseng Supplements. (2006). https://www.consumerlab.com/reviews/Ginseng_Supplements/ginseng/

[3] ConsumerLab.com Product Review of Echinacea Supplements. (2004). http://www.consumerlab.com/reviews/Echinacea/Echinacea/

[4] ConsumerLab.com Product Review of Garlic Supplements. (2006). http://www.consumerlab.com/reviews/Garlic_Supplements/garlic/

[5] ConsumerLab.com Product Review of Memory & Cognition Enhancement Supplements (Ginkgo, Huperzine-A, and Acetyl-L-Carnitine) http://www.consumerlab.com/reviews/Memory_Supplements_Ginkgo_Huperzine_Acetyl-L-Carnitine/GinkgoBiloba/

[6] ConsumerLab.com Product Review of Milk Thistle Supplements. (2009). http://www.consumerlab.com/reviews/Milk_Thistle_Supplements/milkthistle/

[7] ConsumerLab.com Product Review of St. John's *http://www.consumerl* ab.com/reviews/St_Johns_Wort/stjohnswort/

[8] ConsumerLab.com Product Review of Turmeric Supplements. (2008). http://www.consumerlab.com/reviews/Turmeric_Curcumin_Supplements/turmeric/

[9] ConsumerLab.com Product Review of Valerian Supplements. (2006). http://www.consumerlab.com/reviews/Valerian_Supplements/valerian/

[10] ConsumerLab.com Product Review of Joint Health Supplements with Glucosamine, Chondroitin, and/or MSM. (2009). *http://www.consumerlab*.com/reviews/Joint_Supplements_Glucosamine_Chondroitin_and_MSM/jointsup plements/

[11] ConsumerLab.com Asks USP to Adopt Safer Lead Limit for Drugs and

Supplements, December 8, news release. (2008). *http://www.consu* merlab.com/news/USP_Lead_Limit/12_08_2008/

[12] ConsumerLab.com Product Review of Chromium Supplements. (2010). http://www.consumerlab.com/reviews/Chromium/chromium/

[13] Miodovnik, et al. (2009). The U.S. Food and Drug Administration Children's Vitamins Is Based . Environ Health Perspect. July. 117(7). on Outdated 1021-1022. http://www.ncbi.nlm.nih.gov/pmc/articles/PMC2717124/

[14] ConsumerLab.com Product Review of Cholesterol-lowering Supplements. (2010). *http://www.consumerlab.com/reviews/C*holesterol-Lowering_Supplements_Review_Sterols_Policosanol/cholesterol/

[15] ConsumerLab.com Product Review of Supplements for Cancer Prevention (Green Tea, Lycopene and Selenium). (2009). *http://www.consum*erlab.com/reviews/Supplements_for_Cancer_Prevention_Green_Tea_review_Lycope ne_and_Selenium_reviews/cancerprevention/

[16] ConsumerLab.com Product Review of Muscular Enhancement Supplements (Creatine, HMB, Glutamine, BCAAs). (2006). http://www.consumerlab.com/reviews/Muscular_Enhancement_Supplements-Creatine_HMB_Gluatamine_and_BCAAs/creatine/

[17] ConsumerLab.com Product Review of Resveratrol Supplements. (2007). http://www.consumerlab.com/reviews/Resveratrol_Supplements_Including_Red_Wine_Grape_and_Polygonum_Sources/Resveratrol_ Red_Wine/

[18] ConsumerLab.com Product Review of Multivitamin and Multimineral Supplements. (2009). http://www.consumerlab.com/reviews/Multivitamin_Multimineral_Supplements/multivitamins/

[19] ConsumerLab.com Product Review of B Vitamins. (2007). *http://www.c* onsumerlab.com/reviews/B_Vitamins_B-Complexes_Thiamin_Niacin_B-6_B-12_Biotin_and_Folic_Acid/bvitamins/

[20] ConsumerLab.com Archive of Recalls and Warnings *http://www.consum* erlab.com/recalls.asp#Past.

In: Dietary Supplements: What Seniors Need to... ISBN: 978-1-61761-285-5
Editors: Thomas H. Felton

Chapter 4

TESTIMONY OF CHARLES BELL, PROGRAMS DIRECTOR, CONSUMERS UNION, BEFORE THE SENATE SPECIAL COMMITTEE ON AGING, HEARING – "DIETARY SUPPLEMENTS: WHAT SENIORS NEED TO KNOW"

Good afternoon, Chairman Kohl, Ranking Member Corker, and other members of the Committee. Thank you for providing me the opportunity to come before you today. I am Charles Bell, Programs Director for Consumers Union.

Consumers Union is the nonprofit publisher of *Consumer Reports* magazine. Since 1936, our mission at Consumers Union has been to test products, inform the public, and protect consumers. Today I offer this testimony on dietary supplements as part of our consumer protection function.

KEY RECOMMENDATIONS

Consumers and seniors turn to dietary supplements because they think these products will promote health and wellness. They also generally assume that such products are safe for their intended use, and would not be permitted to be sold by the federal government if they were unsafe or posed unreasonable risks to consumers. Unfortunately, in our research and reporting, we have found some very profound and troubling gaps in the system we have today to assure supplement safety. While many dietary supplements, including most vitamins and minerals taken within recommended limits, are generally safe and can have important health benefits for consumers, there is a significant and growing number of highly questionable products that would probably not be allowed on the market if they were subject to rigorous pre-market safety testing.

We believe that Congress should require more rigorous safety standards for dietary supplements. It is very important to ensure that products that are marketed and promoted to advance health are safe, and do not themselves create serious health problems. And, consumers should be assured that the products they buy followed sound manufacturing practices, and are not adulterated or contaminated with heavy metals like lead, or prescription drugs.

Consumers Union supports the Dietary Supplement Safety Act of 2010 (S 3002), that would strengthen public oversight of dietary supplements. This bill includes provisions for manufacturer registration, mandatory recall authority, and improved reporting of non-serious adverse events. We believe that the principles incorporated in this legislation would give regulators better tools for protecting the public, and help move us to a safer marketplace.

The elements of a strong, preventive safety system that we favor include the following:

- **Mandatory Manufacturer Registration Requirements**. The GAO has reported that FDA has relatively little information on the companies it is expected to regulate and oversee. All dietary supplement manufacturing, processing and holding facilities should be required to register annually with the Secretary of Health and Human Services, so that the FDA will know who is making dietary supplements, which products the companies manufacture, and which ingredients the product contain. This will ensure better communication between manufacturers and safety officials, and facilitate swift action in the event of serious adverse events, warnings and safety recalls.
- **Mandatory Recall Authority for the FDA**. The FDA must have the necessary authority to swiftly recall unsafe products that pose risks to consumers.
- **Increased Safety Requirements for Products.** While we favor encouraging the FDA to publish new guidelines for new dietary ingredients, we also believe that the burden of proof for demonstrating

that a supplement does not present a "significant or unreasonable risk" should be placed on manufacturers to establish that supplements are safe before they are sold. In that sense, we are also concerned about existing products that are "grandfathered in" that have not been rigorously tested or reviewed for safety. We support creation of a regulatory review process that would prioritize and address existing hazards in the supplements marketplace, such as the unsafe supplements we have identified that continue to be widely sold in stores and the internet. Products that pose unreasonable risks to consumers are swiftly removed by manufacturers and the FDA.

- **Better Information for Consumers and Medical Providers.** Labels of dietary supplements should clearly indicate what and how much is in the package, and provide explicit warning of possible adverse effects, including herb-drug interactions. FDA should also provide better, real-time information to consumers, medical providers and the public on emerging supplement hazards and adverse event reports, through better use of data systems like the Poison Control Centers and research by independent safety experts.
- **More Comprehensive Reporting of Adverse Events.** Since 2007, manufacturers have been required to report serious, generally life-threatening events to the FDA within 15 days. However, there is much more adverse event information and consumer complaints that are received by manufacturers that should be reported to FDA on an annual basis, or more frequently if possible. Given that our safety system is, in effect, a "post-marketing system," improving the flow of information about adverse events is critical for detecting potential safety hazards, including problems related to contamination and drug interactions.
- **Quality Assurance for Imported Ingredients.** Congress should investigate further ways to assure the safety and quality of supplements manufactured overseas, including expanding funding, oversight resources, investigation and enforcement to assure the safety of imported supplement ingredients.
- **Expanded Efforts to Reduce and Eliminate Supplement Contamination.** Efforts to implement safe manufacturing and production practices should be accelerated, with vigorous oversight by FDA. Dietary supplements should be consistently low in heavy metals and other forms of chemical or mineral contamination, and there should be zero tolerance for prescription drug contamination.

- **Expanded Resources for FDA.** FDA must be provided with sufficient funding and personnel resources to implement a preventive safety system and accomplish its critically important supplement safety mission, by increasing oversight, inspections and enforcement.

SENIOR USE OF DIETARY SUPPLEMENTS

Americans spend an estimated $20-30 billion on dietary supplements annually, and estimates of consumer use of supplements range from 10% to 52% of the overall population.[1] A national telephone survey published in JAMA in 2002 found that vitamins were taken by 40% of respondents, and that herbals and supplements were taken by 14% of those surveyed. Among prescription drug users, 16% also took a supplement.[2]

Findings from several sources suggest that dietary supplement use generally increases with age.

- An internet survey carried out by Mintel in May 2009 found that 67% of 55 to 64 year-olds, and 75% of consumers over the age of 65, report use of regular vitamin supplements, compared with 50% of 45 to 54 year-olds reporting vitamin supplement use, and reported an average use of 52% for the population as a whole.[3]
- According to a recent article published in Nutriceuticals World, consumers between the ages of 65 and 74 are the most frequent users of dietary supplements.
  "…[S]eniors are twice as likely as any other age group to take fish oil/omega 3s, vitamin E, and calcium supplements; they are also heavy users of vitamin C, B12 and B complex, and to a lesser extent antioxidants and herbals."[4]
- According to a survey published in JAMA in 2006, 49% of Americans aged 57 to 85 used a dietary supplement. 52% of seniors reported using supplements concurrently with prescription drugs.[5]

What Seniors and Consumers Need to Know about Dietary Supplements

Many dietary supplements, including most vitamins and minerals taken within recommended limits, are generally safe and can have important health benefits for consumers. However, a significant and growing number of highly questionable products are entering the market that would probably would fail rigorous pre-market safety testing.

Consumers need to be aware that there are significant unresolved safety problems with dietary supplements. Dietary supplements may interact with other prescription drugs, over-the-counter drugs and supplements they are currently taking. We urge all consumers to discuss the use of supplements with their physicians and medical providers prior to initiating use of these products. Further we urge consumers to do their homework, and carefully consider the medical evidence that supports or advises against the use of particular products, by consulting reputable web sites, such as those operated by the National Institutes of Health Office of Dietary Supplements and the FDA.

Dietary supplement products are sold in the same stream of commerce as approved over-the-counter products, and consumers often assume that if they were not safe, the government would not permit them to be sold.

For example, in an October 2002 nationwide Harris Poll of 1,010 adults, 59 percent of respondents said they believed that supplements must be approved by a government agency before they can be sold to the public. Sixty-eight percent said the government requires warning labels on supplements' potential side effects or dangers. Fifty-five percent said supplement manufacturers can't make safety claims without solid scientific support.

Unfortunately, the respondents in this poll are incorrect. None of those widely expected protections exist for dietary supplements—they exist only for prescription and over-the-counter medicines. With respect to testing for hazards, before approval, drugs must be proved effective, with an acceptable safety profile, by means of lab research and rigorous human clinical trials involving a minimum of several thousand people, and several years. In contrast, supplement manufacturers can introduce new products without any testing for safety and efficacy. The maker's only current obligation is to send the FDA a copy of the language on the label.

Drug labels and package inserts must mention all possible adverse effects and interactions. But supplement makers do not have to put safety warnings on the labels, even for products with known serious hazards. With respect to post-surveillance monitoring, drug companies are required by law to tell the FDA about any reports of product-related adverse events that they receive from any source. Almost every year, drugs are removed from the market based on safety risks that first surfaced in those reports.

By contrast, supplement makers were only recently required to report serious adverse events to FDA, beginning at the end of 2007, and many other reports and complaints received by manufacturers are not required to be reported. As a result, FDA has only partial information about consumer safety problems arising from supplement use. In 2001, the HHS Inspector General reported that the FDA Medwatch system was an "inadequate safety valve" for detecting safety problems with dietary supplements, and many of the problems identified by the HHS, the GAO and other agencies continue to this day.

Under DSHEA, the burden of proof for removing unsafe products has been inappropriately shifted from manufacturers to government. As former FDA director David Kessler has stated, "Congress put the FDA in the position of being able to act only after the fact and after substantial harm has already occurred."

In the aftermath of DSHEA, unsafe dietary supplement products can remain on the market for many years, in the same stream of commerce as products approved by the FDA as safe and effective for their intended use. Further, new dietary supplement products can be introduced overnight that contain novel, untested ingredients and/or novel combinations of new and/or existing supplement ingredients. Health providers and public health authorities typically receive little pre-market or post-market information about how such products may affect human health, and interact with medicines that patients are already taking.

Even where serious safety problems are documented, it is difficult for the FDA to take prompt action to protect consumers. Unless the FDA meets a high standard of proof that a dietary supplement creates "a significant or unreasonable risk," it cannot ban it. Over the last 16 years, the FDA has typically relied on warnings and voluntary compliance to address supplement hazards, allowing many dangerous products to remain on the market.

UNSAFE SUPPLEMENTS CAN REMAIN ON THE MARKET FOR MANY YEARS

Consumer Reports periodically publishes lists of unsafe supplements that we urge our readers to avoid. Unfortunately, these unsafe products do not quickly disappear from the marketplace, but continue to be widely sold through retail stores and the internet. Consumers and seniors are being put at risk by an inadequate safety system that does not move swiftly to remove dangerous products from the marketplace.

In 1995, *Consumer Reports* magazine published a list of five supplements that according to the FDA can cause serious harm to consumers--ephedra, chaparral, comfrey, lobelia, and yohimbe. Nine years later, on April 12, 2004ephedra was finally removed from the marketplace, many years after the FDA first received reports of serious consumer health problems, including deaths and disabling injuries. But the other four supplements are still being marketed and sold in retail stores and on the internet.

In May 2004, *Consumer Reports* published an updated list of 12 hazardous dietary supplements, including the four herbs named in the 1995 report, that are too dangerous to be on the market according to government warnings, adverse-event reports, and medical experts.

These "dirty dozen" unsafe supplements, which *CR* easily purchased in stores and online also included aristolochia, an herb conclusively linked to kidney failure and cancer; germander, and kava, which are known or likely causes of liver failure, and bitter orange, a herbal stimulant being marketed as a substitute for ephedra. We pointed out that the potentially dangerous effects of most of these products have been known for more than a decade, and at least five of them were banned in Asia, Europe, or Canada.

The 2004 *Consumer Reports* article described the case of Beverly Hames, who went to an acupuncturist in 1992 seeking a “safe, natural” treatment for an aching back. She obtained a selection of Chinese herbal products, at least five of which were later found to contain aristolochic acid. By mid-1994, she had symptoms of kidney failure, and in 1996 she underwent a kidney transplant. She must take anti-rejection drugs for life. The herbs’ distributor said his Chinese suppliers had substituted Aristolochia for another herb without his knowledge. “I was told that these herbs are safe, they're natural and they've been used for hundreds of years," Hames said. “I went from a perfectly healthy person to kidney failure in a very short period of time."

In January 2008, we updated our list again, and added three additional supplements that we believe pose significant hazards to consumers: cesium, which poses risks of fainting and abnormal heart rhythms; graviola, which has been linked to reports of a nerve disorder similar to Parkinson's disease; and colloidal silver, which can cause kidney damage and irreversible skin discoloration.

While we believe that all of the supplements named in our 1995, 2004 and 2008 reports should be removed from the marketplace immediately, we believe it would be a serious mistake to attempt to address the crisis in supplement safety only on an ad-hoc, substance-by-substance basis. Consumers need effective safety and quality assurance that the supplements they take are safe and effective for their intended use. The type of serious adverse reactions that we see reported for many products, such as heart arrhythmias, liver and kidney damage, strokes and even death, are not the normal sort of surprise that one would expect to find from purchasing a dietary supplement at the corner pharmacy or the internet.

The fact is, with some 30,000 or more dietary supplement products in the marketplace, and an additional 1,000 products entering every year, no one really knows the full number of hazardous products that may be out there. The consumer interest also requires establishment of an effective preventive safety system that includes manufacturer registration, pre-market safety evaluation, mandatory reporting for the full range adverse events, improved oversight of manufacturing practices, and increased FDA regulatory authority to take prompt action against known and emerging hazards.

New Weight-Loss Products Marketed as "Ephedra-Free" May Still Be Unsafe

Many companies have developed new weight-loss supplements that are being marketed as "ephedra-free," which many consumers may assume are safe for consumer use. But as Dr. Paul Coates of the National Institute of Health's Office of Dietary Supplements has warned, "The fact that a dietary supplement is ephedra-free is not a indication of its safety."[6]

Consumers spend some $17.7 billion for dietary and weight-loss supplements each year, and it has been projected that this market grows at 6-7% per year.[7] Because of safety concerns, *Consumer Reports* urges consumers to avoid all dietary supplements marketed for weight loss, because many contain dangerous stimulants and high levels of caffeine.

Many weight loss supplements that are being marketed as "ephedra-free" contain bitter orange. Bitter orange is derived from the Seville orange and has the botanical name citrus aurantium. It appears in some foods, including orange marmalades. In dietary supplements, it appears in a concentrated form, and its active ingredient—synephrine—mimics the effects of ephedra. Synephrine stimulates the cardiovascular system, raises the heart rate, raises blood pressure, and stimulates the central nervous system. While its use has been studied in animals, there have been few studies involving human subjects.

In its May 2004 article, *Consumer Reports* profiled a 21-year-old college student studying for finals who took weight loss supplements containing bitter orange, believing they were safe because they were labeled as "ephedra-free." After three weeks of taking the product, she experienced a seizure. Her neurologist told her that the bitter orange in the supplement product was a likely cause. Since discontinuing use of the supplement, she has not experienced any more seizures.

Multi-Ingredient Dietary Supplements May Pose Significant Hazards

Many weight-loss and body-building supplements, and also supplements marketed for enhancing sexual capacity, contain multiple herbal ingredients, extracts, caffeine, green tea and other ingredients. Many of these ingredients are also marketed as "proprietary blends" so the consumer does not necessarily know how much of each ingredient the product contains, and potential hazards it poses.

In general, little is known about how multiple herbal ingredients, extracts and compounds interact together. Further, these products often contain ingredients that *Consumer Reports* has singled out for concern, including bitter orange, yohimbe, and high levels of caffeine. In a pilot project carried out in California, researchers found that nearly half of reports to local poison control centers involved multi-component supplements containing caffeine.[8] Again, *Consumer Reports* urges consumers to avoid such multi-component weight-loss supplements, both because they may contain high levels of caffeine and other untested ingredients, and there is a lack of medical research to substantiate either their safety or efficacy for the marketed use.

Post-Marketing Surveillance of Dietary Supplements is "an Inadequate Safety Valve"

In April 2001, the Office of Inspector General at the Department of Health and Human Services concluded that the FDA's adverse event reporting system was "an inadequate safety valve" because of inadequate authority and organizational capacity to collect and take action on adverse event reports. The report noted that in contrast to requirements for monograph drugs and new drug application (NDA) drugs, manufacturers of dietary supplements are not required to register their companies or their products with the FDA. As a result, the FDA does not have a list of supplement products and ingredients when it receives an adverse event report. The Inspector General found that FDA was unable to determine the ingredients for 32 percent of products mentioned in adverse event reports (AERs). It also lacked product labels for 77 percent of the products mentioned in the AERs, and product samples for 69 percent of products that it requested. For products referenced in the AERs, the FDA was unable to determine the manufacturer for 32 percent of the products, and the city and state for 71 percent of manufacturers.

As discussed above, many consumers are surprised to learn the government does not currently evaluate the safety of dietary supplements before they are sold. This situation poses a serious risk to public health, and amounts to a vast, uncontrolled clinical trial on an unsuspecting public. Mr. Joseph Levitt, Esq., Director of the FDA's Center for Food Safety and Applied Nutrition, testified in Congress in March 2001 that the current "regulation of dietary supplements is, for the most part, a post-marketing program."

Manufacturers Suppressed Information Regarding Dietary Supplement Adverse Events

The safety problems that consumers experienced with ephedra also demonstrated that manufacturers may conceal substantial numbers of consumer complaints regarding their products. Many customer complaints were received by manufacturers that were not forwarded in a timely way to the FDA.

- On August 15, 2002, the Justice Department disclosed that it was investigating whether Metabolife, a major manufacturer and distributor of ephedra products, had made false statements to the FDA regarding the existence of consumer complaints about its products. On the same day, Metabolife announced that it would turn over 13,000 consumer health complaints or "adverse event reports" to the FDA.11 After analyzing the Metabolife adverse events reports, the special investigations division of the House Committee on Government Reform concluded that 2,000 of the 13,000 reports were "significant" effects, including three deaths, 20 heart attacks, 24 strokes, 40 seizures, 465 episodes of chest pains and 966 reports of heart rhythm disturbances.
- Depositions in a lawsuit in San Francisco against E'ola (a Utah-based multilevel-marketing firm) regarding a death allegedly linked to ephedra revealed that the company had received 3,500 customer complaints about one of its ephedra weight-loss products. According to the San Francisco Chronicle, none of the complaints were ever disclosed to the FDA.

On December 22, 2007, mandatory manufacturer reporting of serious adverse events related to dietary supplements went into effect, as a result of provisions included in the Dietary Supplement and Nonprescription Drug Consumer Protection Act, passed in 2006. Manufacturers were directed to report serious events such as serious cardiac, respiratory and gastrointestinal disorders.

However, many so-called non-serious adverse events are not covered by the law that Congress passed, even though this information would help FDA develop a better safety profile for many supplements. But these prominent examples from the past do not inspire confidence that important and significant health impacts arising from the use of herbal supplements will be promptly reported to responsible health authorities under a voluntary reporting system. We remain concerned that the flow of information to FDA needs to be improved to generate better, timely signals of emerging hazards.

Consumers Need Prompt FDA Action and Early Warning about Emerging Hazards

At a minimum, we believe that dietary supplement manufacturers should be required to forward all adverse event reports to FDA on a regular basis. While reporting of non-serious events has been required since the end of 2007, we do not think that the current reporting system gives FDA enough information to trigger timely action against products that pose unreasonable risks to consumers. We are also concerned that consumers do not receive warning about products that pose emerging hazards. Delays in reporting hazards increases potential risks to consumers.

For example, in the case of Hydroxycut, a top-selling weight-loss supplement recalled by FDA on May 1, 2009, the FDA's Medwatch system did not report reported hazards until the product's recall, even though the agency had received six dozen reports of adverse events, including 23 cases of liver toxicity and at least one death.

According to researcher Ano Lobb, a public health consultant who has worked in the past on the Consumer Reports Health Letter, the only warning about Hydroxycut were growing case reports in the medical literature. Lobb also points out that the nation's Poison Control Centers may be detecting 10 times more adverse events related to supplements. The FDA could potentially increase its postmarket surveillance capacity by incorporating the Poison Control Center data, and coordinating with independent researchers who could help provide earlier warning of supplement hazards.[9]

Seniors Need to be Aware of the Serious Potential Risks of Interactions between Prescription Drugs and Dietary Supplements

Consumers may also experience safety problems with dietary supplements because of potential interactions with existing health conditions, such as diabetes, coronary problems or hypertension, and with other prescription or over-the counter medications they are currently taking.

As noted above, according to a survey published in JAMA in 2006, 49% of Americans aged 57 to 85 used a dietary supplement. 52% of seniors reported using supplements concurrently with prescription drugs.[10] It is very important for seniors to understand that prescription drugs may interact in many complex ways with other prescription drugs, over-the-counter drugs and dietary supplements. The bottom line is that patients and physicians need to discuss the specific products that the consumer is taking, to avoid adverse interactions and ensure that prescribed treatments will be effective.

Few clinical studies have systematically assessed potential interactions between supplements and medications, and many potential concerns have been reported. Depending on the combination of prescription drugs, OTC drugs and supplements the consumer may be taking, the effectiveness of intended treatments may be reduced, and the patient may be put at minor or serious risk in a wide range of other ways.

In particular, herbal remedies can interact dangerously with medications. In the January 2007 issue of Consumer Reports Health, we published an article on "Risky herb-drug combos" that listed potential interactions with nine top selling herbal supplements and common prescription drugs. Potential effects fall into four categories:

1. reduced drug efficacy
2. increased chance of drug side effects
3. potentially dangerous increases in drug efficacy
4. and potentially dangerous rise in drug efficacy AND increased chance of side effects.

As an example, ginkgo biloba, a popular supplement taken to enhance memory taken by as many as 11 million Americans, may reduce platelets in the blood, and make it more difficult for the blood to clot. This can cause excessive bleeding, and in some cases strokes. Because of the potential complications with surgical procedures, Dr. John Neeld, the president of the American Society of Anesthesiologists, advises consumers to discontinue the use of herbal medicine at least 2 to 3 weeks prior to surgery.

A recent article published in the Journal of the American College of Cardiology provides a detailed description of potential interactions for herbal interactions for patients who have cardiovascular diseases. The article lists 27 commonly sold herbal products that patients with such diseases may need to avoid, and points out that the evidence for safety and efficacy for many of these products is scant. The article advises physicians to carefully question patients about supplement use, especially elderly patients who may be at higher risk.[11]

According to Dr. Arthur Grollman, professor of medicine and pharmacy-ological sciences at the State University of New York at Stony Brook:

> Interactions between herbal products and prescription or over-the-counter drugs constitutes one of the greatest risks posed by the used of botanical medicines. Botanical medicines can act through a variety of mechanisms to alter the actions and metabolism of prescription and OTC drugs.... In fact, serious adverse effects have been reported in patients taking cyclosporine or antiretroviral agents when they added St. John's wort, which caused blood levels of their life-saving drug to fall to amounts that were no longer therapeutic.
>
> The extent of herb-drug interactions is unclear, but its potential magnitude can be judged by a recent survey of medication use in the U.S. A recent survey found that among individuals over 18 years of age, 50% took at least one prescription drug during the preceding week. Among women over 65 years or older, 23% took at least five prescription drugs. 16% of those taking prescription drugs also took an herbal supplement. Thus, many Americans unknowingly risk therapeutic failures or adverse effects due to herb-drug interactions, especially older individuals who take multiple medications for chronic diseases.[12]

For these reasons, *Consumer Reports* recommends that consumers discuss the use of all dietary supplements with their physicians or health providers prior to taking them, to guard against the possibility of adverse health effects or drug reactions. The American Society of Anesthesiologists reported several years ago that as many as seven in 10 consumers do not discuss the use of supplements with their doctor. Ensuring open channels of communication between physicians and patients about supplement use and potential drug-supplement interactions is critical for promoting and maintaining good health.

Contamination of Dietary Supplements with Prescription Drugs and Heavy Metals

From January through September 2007, the FDA issued nine "safety alerts" warning consumers to stop using 13 brands marketed as supplements, because FDA testing found that they contained prescription medications. Nine concealed erectile-dysfunction drugs such as sildenafil (Viagra) or tadalafil (Cialis), three harbored lovastatin (Mevacor), a prescription drug for high chloresterol; and one, sibutramine (Meridia), a weight loss drug. These products unknowingly put consumers at risk of pharmaceutical side effects and potential drug interactions.

In August 2009, the FDA discovered more than 140 products, most of them labeled as dietary supplements, that were contaminated with prescription drugs. In some cases, the level of the prescription weight loss drug sibutramine was up to three times the maximum recommended daily drug dose.

On May 3, 2010, the Food and Drug Administration warned consumers against using Vita Breath, after a patient with lead poisoning reported using the supplement plus two other herbal products. The New York City Department of Health and Mental Hygiene alerted the FDA to the case of lead poisoning. When that agency tested Vita Breath, it found the drug contained 1,100 parts per million of lead, that's 10,000 times higher than the FDA's maximum allowable lead levels for candy.

Vita Breath, which is manufactured by American Herbal Lab in California, is sold at health fairs and on the internet. People who have taken Vita Breath should talk to their health care provider about getting their lead levels tested. The FDA is currently analyzing samples of the dietary supplement, and working with New York and California officials to further investigate the product.

Acute lead poisoning symptoms can include abdominal pain, muscle weakness, nausea, vomiting, diarrhea, weight loss and bloody or decreased urinary output. Children are particularly vulnerable to lead poisoning. Also note that people with high levels of lead in their blood may show no symptoms, but the condition can still damage the nervous system and internal organs.

According to an article by Dr. Peter Cohen in the New England Journal of Medicine, such reports represent only the fraction of the contaminated supplements that are probably present in the marketplace. Dr. Cohen points out the unscrupulous manufacturers have made it more difficult for the FDA to detect the contamination by modifying the original chemical structure of the drug to elude testing. According to the article, many of the contaminated products found to date were made in China, Brazil and other countries.[13]

Consumers Union is concerned that FDA is not providing adequate oversight of supplement contamination problems. We need to assure consumers that dietary supplements are consistently low in heavy metals and other forms of chemical or mineral contamination, and we should have zero tolerance for prescription drug contamination. At a minimum, we believe that products should not exceed U.S. Pharmacopeia limits for lead and other heavy metals. Because consumers do not expect to encounter heavy metal contamination in supplements, and many consumers may take multiple supplements or multiple doses of supplements, additional oversight may be needed to reduce hazards and warn consumers about unexpected health risks.

NEW UNTESTED NANO-INGREDIENTS IN SUPPLEMENTS

In 2009, the Project on Emerging Nanotechnologies reported that 44 dietary supplement products that claim to contain nano-particles were on the market. Yet the FDA has little information about such products, and there are serious questions about whether such products are safe for consumers to use.[14]

"It is not clear that the supplement industry is conducting the rigorous testing needed either to understand the effects of nanoscale ingredients in its products or to back up the product claims. This means that consumers are potentially exposed to unknown risks that should be balanced with the possible benefits of taking these supplements," says David Rejeski, PEN's director.

The Project has issued a report entitled "A Hard Pill to Swallow: Barriers to Effective Regulation of Dietary Supplements Containing Nanoparticles."

According to the Report's Executive Summary:

The FDA's ability to regulate the safety of dietary supplements using nanomaterials is severely limited by lack of information, lack of resources and the agency's lack of statutory authority in certain critical areas. Three main problems need to be addressed:

1. FDA does not have the capacity to identify nano-based dietary supplements that are being developed and marketed, unless manufacturers submit to the pre-market notification process for new dietary ingredients.
2. To the extent that FDA is aware of nano-based dietary supplements, it has little regulatory authority over them.
3. Even if it were granted increased regulatory authority, FDA lacks the scientific expertise and resources to effectively regulate nanomaterials in supplements.

The report recommends that Congress adopt legislation granting FDA the authority to collect additional information about those supplement products containing nano-particles, and ensure that they are tested for their effects on human health.

"Such legislation should prohibit the sale of new dietary supplements made with nanotechnology until they have been demonstrated to be safe, and it should provide FDA with sufficient resources to regulate these products," according to the report. "...Until Congress acts, consumers who take dietary supplements containing engineered nanoparticles will be at additional, unknowable and potentially serious risk."[15]

Quality Assurance for Imported Ingredients

Another important concern for seniors and consumers is assuring the quality of imported ingredients that are used in dietary supplements. These concerns were recently highlighted by a report issued by the U.S.-China Economic and Security Review Commission. NSD Bio Group LLC, a research group under contract to the Commission, reported in April that there are a variety of potential concerns regarding the expanded sourcing of pharmaceutical and dietary supplement products and ingredients from China.[16]

The report comes in the wake of health concerns raised by unsafe raw materials discovered in imported products from China. There have been numerous recalls and warning issued by US firms in the last several years in relation due to health and safety concerns about products and ingredients imported from China. These have included heparin (a blood thinner widely used by kidney-dialysis and post-surgical patients to prevent blood clots), and wheat gluten (corrupted with the chemical melamine). Melamine was found in animal feed and pet food in the US 2007, and dairy products and infant formula in China in 2008.

The Commission report examines the potential health and safety impacts of Chinese-sourced ingredients used in the production and supply of pharmaceutical products, dietary and nutritional supplements. China is now the largest bulk drug manufacturing and exporter in the world, and has emerged as America's number one pharmaceutical trade partner. China is also the number one producer of Acetominophen and many other commonly used over-the-counter cold and allergy medications.

The report also notes the huge and growing size of the US market for dietary and nutritional supplements, and points out that many US nutrition supply companies are either based in China or do extensive sourcing there.

"China has come to dominate the vitamin raw material market over the last decade, controlling approximately one third of the world's vitamin production," according to the report. For example, China now supplies 92% of the vitamin C, 65% of vitamin B, and 40% of vitamin E raw materials imported into the U.S.

Obviously, these concerns are not just limited to China. US health and safety officials must assure the safety of all imported products that are used in the US, particularly food, drugs and supplements, regardless of the country of origin. As foreign trading partners play a larger role in supplying nutritional supplements and materials for their production, there is an urgent need for greater public oversight to assure the quality of imported products and ingredients.

While the FDA has recently launched new initiatives to expand its Foreign Drug Inspection Program and has stationed a handful of inspectors in China, we are concerned that current oversight capacity and process is grossly inadequate for the task of policing such a diverse array and large volume of imported products and ingredients. Even if we were to just take the sourcing and manufacture of herbal products alone, it does not appear that FDA has either the funding or the staff resources to adequately assure the safe sourcing and supply of such ingredients. As an example, we would cite continuing reports of contamination of herbal supplements with prescription drugs and heavy metals, and also the problems related to the Chinese herb aristolochia, which we reported about in our May 2004 Consumer Reports article.

Consumers and seniors need to be assured that the oversight processes we have in place will prevent serious safety problems, and enable swift regulatory action and effective recalls when problems are detected and found. Because of the recent surge in product warnings and recalls, this is an urgent issue that must be addressed swiftly. We urge Congress to investigate problems and issues related to sourcing of dietary supplement ingredients from China and other exporting nations, and work rapidly to modernize the regulatory infrastructure to address this new challenge.

Recommendations

As a nation, we stand at a crossroads regarding dietary supplement safety. Consumers turn to dietary supplements because they think these products will promote health and wellness. It is very important to ensure that these products are safe and do not themselves create serious health problems. Consumers who take supplements should not be test animals for highly questionable products that have not been sufficiently tested by their manufacturers prior to coming to market.

For the last sixteen years, consumers have borne the unacceptable risks and consequences of system that allows untested supplements to be aggressively marketed and sold, with no prior safety testing and evaluation. This situation unfairly shifts the burden of proof to demonstrate supplements are safe before they can be sold from manufacturers to the government, and externalizes the costs and risks of that policy onto consumers and the health system.

We believe that Congress should make steady and sure progress toward developing a sensible preventive safety system that ensures that dietary supplement products are reviewed for safety prior to marketing and sale.

Consumers Union supports the Dietary Supplement Safety Act of 2010 (S 3002), that would strengthen public oversight of dietary supplements. This bill includes provisions for manufacturer registration, mandatory recall authority, improved reporting of non-serious adverse events. We believe that the principles incorporated in this legislation would give regulators better tools for protecting the public, and help move us to a safer marketplace

The elements of a strong, preventive safety system that we favor include the following:

- **Mandatory Manufacturer Registration Requirements**. The GAO has reported that FDA has relatively little information on the companies it is expected to regulate and oversee. All dietary supplement manufacturing, processing and holding facilities should be required to register annually with the Secretary of Health and Human Services, so that the FDA will know who is making dietary supplements, which products the companies manufacture, and which ingredients the product contain. This will ensure better communication between manufacturers and safety officials, and facilitate swift action in the event of serious adverse events, warnings and safety recalls.
- **Mandatory Recall Authority for the FDA**. The FDA must have the necessary authority to swiftly recall unsafe products that pose risks to consumers.
- **Increased Safety Requirements for Products.** While we favor encouraging the FDA to publish new guidelines for new dietary ingredients, we also believe that the burden of proof for demonstrating that a supplement does not present a "significant or unreasonable risk"

should be placed on manufacturers to establish that supplements are safe before they are sold. In that sense, we are also concerned about existing products that are "grandfathered in" that have not been rigorously tested or reviewed for safety. We support creation of a regulatory review process that would prioritize and address existing hazards in the supplements marketplace, such as the unsafe supplements we have identified that continue to be widely sold in stores and the internet. Products that pose unreasonable risks to consumers are swiftly removed by manufacturers and the FDA.

- **Better Information for Consumers and Medical Providers.** Labels of dietary supplements should clearly indicate what and how much is in the package, and provide explicit warning of possible adverse effects, including herb-drug interactions. FDA should also provide better, real-time information to consumers, medical providers and the public on emerging supplement hazards and adverse event reports, through better use of data systems like the Poison Control Centers and research by independent safety experts.
- **More Comprehensive Reporting of Adverse Events.** Since 2007, manufacturers have been required to report serious, generally life-threatening events to the FDA within 15 days. However, there is much more adverse event information and consumer complaints that are received by manufacturers that should be reported to FDA on an annual basis, or more frequently if possible. Given that our safety system is, in effect, a "post-marketing system," improving the flow of information about adverse events is critical for detecting potential safety hazards, including problems related to contamination and drug interactions.
- **Quality Assurance for Imported Ingredients.** Congress should investigate further ways to assure the safety and quality of supplements manufactured overseas, including expanding funding, oversight resources, investigation and enforcement to assure the safety of imported supplement ingredients.
- **Expanded Efforts to Reduce and Eliminate Supplement Contamination.** Efforts to implement safe manufacturing and production practices should be accelerated, with vigorous oversight by FDA. Dietary supplements should be consistently low in heavy metals and other forms of chemical or mineral contamination, and there should be zero tolerance for prescription drug contamination.

- **Expanded Resources for FDA.** FDA must be provided with sufficient funding and personnel resources to implement a preventive safety system and accomplish its critically important supplement safety mission, by increasing oversight, inspections and enforcement.

CONCLUSION

Mr. Chairman, Members of the Committee, thank you very much for the opportunity to testify here today about this critically important consumer protection issue. We thank you for your efforts to protect consumers in these tough economic times, and look forward to working with you as you move forward in addressing these issues.

End Notes

[1] Gardiner, P., Sarma, DN, Low Dog T, Barret ML, Chavez ML, Mahady GB, Marples RJ, Giancaspro GI. The state of dietary adverse event reporting in the United States. Pharmacoepidem Drug Safety, 2008: 17(10): 962-970. See also: Tachjian A, Maria V, Jahangir A. Use of Herbal Products and Potential Interactions in Patients with Cardiovascular Diseases. Journal of the American College of Cardiology, 2/9/10, Vol 55, No. 6 2010, 515-25.

[2] Kaufman DW, Kelly JP, Roseberg L, Andersen TE, Mitchael AA. Recent Patterns of Medication Use in the Ambulatory Adult Population of the U.S.: The Slone Survey. JAMA 1/16/02 Vol 287, No. 3, 337-344.

[3] Mintel, "Functional Foods – US," August 2009. Base: 2,000 Internet users aged 18+.

[4] "Up and coming markets: an ounce of prevention equals a pound of cure," Nutraceuticals World, September 2009.

[5] Dima M. Qato, PharmD, MPH; G. Caleb Alexander, MD, MS; Rena M. Conti, PhD; Michael Johnson, BA; Phil Schumm, MA; Stacy Tessler Lindau, MD, MAPP. Use of Prescription and Over-the-counter Medications and Dietary Supplements Among Older Adults in the United States. JAMA. 2008;300(24):2867-2878.

[6] Jill Burcum, "Your Health: Ephedra-free products loaded with new herbs of concern," Minneapolis Star Tribune, April 29, 2003.

[7] Tachjian A, Maria V, Jahangir A. Use of Herbal Products and Potential Interactions in Patients with Cardiovascular Diseases. Journal of the American College of Cardiology, 2/9/10, Vol 55, No. 6 2010, 515-25.

[8] Haller C, Kearney T, Bent S, Ko R, Benowitz, N, Olson, K. Dietary Supplement Adverse Events: Report of a One-Year Poison Center Surveillance Project. Journal of Medical Toxicology, June 2008, Vol 4., No. 2.

[9] Lobb A. Enhancing FDA's Post-Market Surveillance of Dietary Supplements: Two Simple Steps to Build Capacity. Journal of Dietary Supplements, 9/21/09, Vol 6(3), 204-210.

[10] Dima M. Qato, PharmD, MPH; G. Caleb Alexander, MD, MS; Rena M. Conti, PhD; Michael Johnson, BA; Phil Schumm, MA; Stacy Tessler Lindau, MD, MAPP. Use of Prescription

and Over-the-counter Medications and Dietary Supplements Among Older Adults in the United States. JAMA. 2008;300(24):2867-2878.

[11] Tachjian A, Maria V, Jahangir A. Use of Herbal Products and Potential Interactions in Patients with Cardiovascular Diseases. Journal of the American College of Cardiology, 2/9/10, Vol 55, No. 6 2010, 515-25.

[12] Grollman, Arthur, MD. Testimony before Senate Commerce Committee hearing on dietary supplements, October 28, 2003.

[13] Cohen P. American Roulette: Contaminated Dietary Supplements, NEJM, 10/7/09, NEJM.org.

[14] Erickson, Britt. "Nanoceuticals?" Chemical and Engineering News, 2/9/09, available at: http://pubs.acs.org/cen/government/87/8706gov3.html

[15] Shultz, William, and Barclay, Lisa. "A Hard Pill to Swallow: Barriers to Effective FDA Regulation of Nanotechnology-Based Dietary Supplements," Project on Emerging Nanotechnologies, January 2009.

[16] NSD Bio Group LLC, "Potential Health and Safety Impacts from Pharmaceuticals and Supplements Containing Chinese-Sourced Ingredients," prepared for the US China Economic and Security Review Commission, April 2010.

In: Dietary Supplements: What Seniors Need to… ISBN: 978-1-61761-285-5
Editors: Thomas H. Felton

Chapter 5

WRITTEN TESTIMONY OF STEVE MISTER, PRESIDENT AND CEO, COUNCIL FOR RESPONSIBLE NUTRITION, BEFORE THE SENATE SPECIAL COMMITTEE ON AGING, HEARING – "DIETARY SUPPLEMENTS: WHAT SENIORS NEED TO KNOW"

The Council for Responsible Nutrition (CRN) appreciates this opportunity to provide testimony to the Senate Special Committee on Aging on behalf of the dietary supplement industry to reassure you and your colleagues, your constituents, and our customers that the dietary supplement industry is committed to manufacturing and marketing high quality, safe and beneficial products that have a valuable and appropriate role in a wellness regimen. This industry is likewise committed to ensuring that consumers receive truthful, accurate and non-misleading information on dietary supplements.

This testimony is submitted on behalf of the five trade associations who collectively represent all segments of the dietary supplement supply chain: ingredient growers, suppliers and processors, manufacturers and retailers. They are: the American Herbal Products Association (AHPA); the Consumer Healthcare Products Association (CHPA); the Council for Responsible Nutrition (CRN); the Natural Products Association (NPA); and the United Natural Products Alliance (UNPA).

These associations share the concerns of the Committee about any bad actors in the industry—those companies, whether they are manufacturers or retailers, that are either unaware of the extensive regulatory framework governing dietary supplements or are willfully breaking the law. At the outset, we want to assure you that our industry condemns adulterated products and false, misleading or deceptive marketing practices—activities engaged in by a very small minority who have damaged the reputation of the responsible industry that comprises the vast majority of supplements sold in this country. The responsible supplement industry has a demonstrated track record of providing high-quality products to its consumers and of active lobbying for stronger regulatory guidelines, for broader implementation of the laws under which our industry operates, and for increased enforcement activity, as well as for adequate funding for the Food and Drug Administration (FDA). Our industry has gone even further—developing educational initiatives for consumers designed to make supplement shoppers more savvy and voluntary self-regulatory programs that address the issues that tarnish our industry and potentially hurt our consumers. The latter include a variety of training programs to inform manufacturers and retailers of the legal requirements and their compliance obligations.

Our industry, like all industries, has its outliers, and we applaud this committee's efforts to shine the spotlight on those activities that break the law. But we would be remiss if we did not put some perspective around these concerns. The great majority of American consumers who take dietary supplements are using safe, high-quality supplements to maintain and improve their healthy lifestyles. Adulterated dietary supplement products remain a small minority of supplement products sold in our country today.

More than 150 million Americans—including many who are extremely passionate about their right to purchase supplements—take dietary supplements each year. We know from market research that a high percentage of our consumers are highly proactive in managing their health, engaging by large measure in other healthy habits such as trying to eat a healthy diet, exercising regularly, visiting their doctors. The data defies the myth that supplement users will forsake other healthy behaviors and put their health solely in the hands of a supplement pill. To the contrary, dietary supplement users are more likely than nonusers to engage in the healthy habits noted above[1]. We also know that among the more than 150 million Americans who use dietary supplements are a high percentage of nine healthcare populations (including physician specialties such as orthopedists, cardiologists, dermatologists and OBGYNs, as well as nurses, nurse practitioners, pharmacists, and registered dietitians) who both personally take and professionally recommend dietary supplements[2]. There are literally millions of shelf units of supplements sold in this country each year—and very few serious adverse events associated with their usage. In 2008 (the last year for which complete data is available), the agency received only 1,025 reports of serious adverse events associated with dietary supplements though it should be noted that these "signals" are not considered by FDA to be evidence that a dietary supplement actually caused the reported event. At the same time, the scientific support continues to grow for the important health benefits of many of our products—products like multivitamins, calcium, fish oil, vitamin D, and more—taken by our core consumers, including the aging and elderly populations.

Every regulated consumer products industry faces the kinds of challenges that the dietary supplement industry faces. By simply enforcing the current law, if the agencies devoted greater focus and had greater resources to fully implement it, these incidents could be further reduced. And when the pending Food Safety legislation (S. 510) is enacted (legislation which our industry supports), there will be additional laws in place—including mandatory recall authority for FDA—to continue to strengthen the regulation of this industry and conventional foods. No matter what the law requires, it is unrealistic to suggest that you would never find a retailer giving bad or illegal advice, or that you could never discover a manufacturing error.

Pharmaceuticals, conventional foods, medical devices and cosmetics—all regulated by FDA—likewise have accidents and rogue players. But our industry has made great strides in the past decade, and we pledge to continue to support reasonable regulation that makes sense for our industry, is not duplicative or contradictory to laws already in place, and that benefits our consumers. However, we will also continue to fight against unnecessarily burdensome regulation that drives up consumer prices, adds unnecessary paperwork and bureaucratic obstacles to market, or restricts truthful information about supplements from reaching consumers—all of which provide no real return or protection for health conscious consumers.

Since the passage of the Dietary Supplement Health & Education Act (DSHEA) in 1994, our industry has come of age, and as we mature, like all industries with growing consumer interest, there are some growing pains. Through the work of the five trade associations, we have fostered an understanding and acceptance, even a desire, among supplement ingredient suppliers, manufacturers and retailers, for strong and enforced regulation—separating those companies who cannot or will not follow the law from those companies who go above and beyond what is legally required. The passage of the 2004 anabolic steroids law, the removal of ephedra, the adverse event reporting law, and the issuance of GMP regulations were all accomplished with the support of the industry associations. As your hearing today points out, clearly, there is more work to be done. As an industry, we are willing to work cooperatively with government, regulators, suppliers, manufacturers, and retailers, as well as consumers, and consumer groups who are willing to partner with us to make certain that the American public has access to the most safe, high-quality dietary supplements the marketplace can offer.

Let us also deal directly with a myth that has been fostered by our critics, perpetuated by the media since 1994, and is widely circulated in the halls of Congress. Many charge that DSHEA de-regulated the industry, stripped FDA of its power over dietary supplements, and rolled back the previous regulation of vitamins. That is simply false. The passage of DSHEA provided FDA with new enforcement authority not previously available:

- It gave FDA the ability to remove from the market supplements that pose a significant or unreasonable risk of injury or illness—a power the agency has used on several occasions since 2000;
- It authorized the creation of GMP regulations distinct for supplements and separate from food GMP regulations;
- It created the imminent hazard to public health standard which allows FDA to remove unsafe products from the marketplace immediately;
- It required notification to FDA for all new dietary ingredients, along with the submission of evidence of reasonable expectation of safety of the ingredient; and,
- It even prescribes that labeling statements about how a dietary supplement will affect the structure or function of the body, so-called "structure/function claims," must be submitted to FDA within 30 days of first use and must be truthful and not misleading with adequate substantiation.

DSHEA made certain that dietary supplements were to be regulated as a category of foods, not drugs. Prior to 1994, on some occasions, FDA regulated supplements as foods; on others, it tried to regulate them as drugs or food additives. But to be clear, FDA never had legal pre-market approval authority for dietary supplements—DSHEA did not change that fact.

The industry would like to address the three areas of highest concern to the Special Committee on Aging. For each area, we will summarize the current legal requirements, demonstrating that the existing law already addresses the concerns that have been raised. Then we will provide information on specific industry programs and voluntary efforts that are also in place to foster compliance, and in many cases, encourage responsible behavior even beyond the requirements of the law. And finally, Senators Harkin and Hatch recently introduced the Dietary Supplement Full Implementation and Enforcement Act of 2010, and we urge this committee to add its support for this legislation as it will propose increased funding for FDA. This legislation will help to ensure that the agency has sufficient focus and resources at its disposal to implement a law—DSHEA—which already provides FDA with ample authority to ensure consumer safety, while still providing consumers access to the products they seek.

PRODUCT QUALITY

Questions have been raised about the quality, purity and potency of dietary supplements and the commitment of supplement manufacturers to produce safe and beneficial products. Three things should be considered here. First, DSHEA requires all dietary supplements to be produced under strict manufacturing conditions to ensure product quality; second, that regulation is being enforced; third, the trade associations are aggressively educating industry of its obligations to ensure product quality.

After years of prodding, pleading and urging from industry, and indeed by some in Congress, FDA issued the final GMP regulations in 2007. Next month, the three-year phase-in of these regulations will be completed and *all* companies finally will be subject to supplement-specific GMPs, nearly 16 years after the passage of DSHEA. Even before the supplement GMPs went into effect for the supplement industry, manufacturers were subject to the requirements of conventional food GMP regulation.

Now, under the GMPs specific to dietary supplements, all manufacturers are required to test every lot of incoming material to confirm the identity of the ingredients. They are required to qualify their vendors so that other aspects of quality—like the purity of the ingredient from contaminants, and the consistency of the material—are assured. These rules mandate training of personnel, master batch records and production logs, calibration of equipment and measuring devices, cleanliness of the work environment to prevent cross contamination, and testing of finished products against label claim, just to name a few. While no law can provide complete assurance against mishaps, these regulations, when fully implemented will give consumers more confidence than ever in the quality of supplements.

To its credit, after issuance of the GMPs and in the face of competing resource needs, FDA has pursued an aggressive industry education effort to be sure supplement companies understand their obligations under the new regulations. The agency has already conducted numerous inspections under the new GMPs, and the industry is encouraged that FDA has announced a robust agenda of inspections in the coming year. And while the discovery of violations is not a positive development, the issuance within the last month of a warning letter on GMP compliance issues that resulted from an inspection signals that FDA has the tools available to insist that industry members comply with the rules. What the agency needs is more resources to put sufficient, well-trained inspectors in the field.

The collective efforts of all five industry trade associations further demonstrate the commitment of this industry to full implementation of the GMPs. Over the past three years, our organizations have hosted over 25 well-attended educational events for industry to acquaint manufacturers with the new GMP rule and explore the specific requirements it imposes. Our efforts range from webinars and conference calls with industry and FDA representatives, to trade show conferences and all-day symposia, as well as creating manuals, chapters and by-lined articles on the GMPs to companies offering personalized seminars.

The trade associations have also developed the Standardized Information for Dietary Ingredients protocol, or "SIDI," for short. This collective effort, across all five associations, has helped to standardize the communications between ingredient suppliers and manufacturers so that manufacturers can compare competing ingredients, obtain all relevant information documentation about the quality of ingredients, and make smarter purchasing decisions. That effort has expanded to produce another voluntary guideline that prescribes best practices for developing the Certificate of Analysis that accompanies each lot of raw material shipped to a manufacturer—and even more industry-endorsed, voluntary guidelines are planned.

The Natural Products Association has developed the GMP Certification program, one of several opportunities for manufacturers to undergo rigorous inspection and receive certification of their products. Manufacturers voluntarily permit third party auditors to inspect their facilities and test their products in hopes of receiving a seal of approval for their labels. Over 60 companies have participated in this program. NPA's TruLabel program randomly selects products from retail shelves and tests their contents for conformance with the label. If a product is determined to be out of conformance, the company is notified and asked to take corrective action.

The United Natural Products Alliance has offered numerous GMP and quality management seminars for industry executives in conjunction with FDA, the University of Mississippi, the United States Pharmacopeia, AOAC International and NSF International. Such training programs provide state of the art instruction on analytical methods, vendor qualification, certificates of analysis, botanical identification and other important technical subjects. (See www.unpa.com for all seminar programs.)

Do all these efforts assure with 100% certainty that a laboratory will never find a product on a store shelf that doesn't meet the GMPs? Of course not. But more than ever, dietary supplement manufacturers have every incentive to produce the best quality products, and real sanctions in place if they don't.

Related to the issue of quality, are persistent questions about the safety of some dietary ingredients. Under DSHEA, dietary supplement ingredients already on the market in the United States as of October 1994 were "grandfathered," in the same way the 1958 food additive amendments to the FDCA "grandfathered" as safe hundreds of substances already being used in foods at the time. DSHEA also established a premarket notification procedure that requires manufacturers who use new ingredients in dietary supplements after 1994 to provide a notification to FDA that sets forth the basis for considering the ingredient to be "reasonably expected to be safe," and there is clear authority in DSHEA for FDA to declare a supplement adulterated if it contains a new dietary ingredient for which an NDI notification was not filed. FDA has been receiving these notifications on a regular basis since the passage of DSHEA and has been giving them serious attention. But the agency has objected to about 70% of the more than 500 notifications it has received.

To assist industry members in filing NDI notices, the American Herbal Products Association created an NDI Database designed to ease access to and understanding of the notifications submitted to FDA. The searchable database allows companies to easily locate individual notifications by searching for key terms that include the generic and brand name of the NDI itself and the Latin name (genus) of herbal NDIs, as well as the name of the submitting firm or the report number assigned by FDA.

What is needed, though, to increase success in filing NDI notifications, is a formal guidance from FDA that explains clearly the agency's views on what constitutes a new dietary ingredient versus a grandfathered one and provides instruction on how firms can establish the reasonable expectation of safety from the evidence they provide. Industry has been asking for this guidance for years and FDA has been promising it, but to date, it has not been issued.

PRODUCT ADVERTISING AND LABELING CLAIMS

This Committee has also raised questions about the advertising and marketing of dietary supplements, inquiring whether there is adequate protection for consumers from false or misleading advertising. As with the product quality issue, the answers begin in the plain language of the statute. DSHEA expressly requires that all labeling claims must be truthful, not misleading, and substantiated with adequate evidence. In addition, DSHEA sets clear boundaries on permissible claims for supplements. Any claim to treat, prevent, mitigate or cure a disease is not permitted, and the statute provides that such claims render the product an unapproved new drug, subject to various civil and criminal penalties. Health claims—those that make an association between a dietary ingredient and the reduction of risk of a disease, such as calcium's ability to reduce the risk of osteoporosis—require the approval of FDA based on significant scientific agreement. Even structure/function claims that do not require the approval of FDA, nevertheless are required by the statute to be submitted to FDA within 30 days of the first use, giving the agency oversight for the kinds of claims that are made.

The Federal Trade Commission (FTC), not FDA, has jurisdiction over dietary supplement advertising. The general standards for consumer advertising apply to supplement claims, but FTC has stated that it "gives great deference to an FDA determination of whether there is adequate support for a health claim. Furthermore, FTC and FDA will generally arrive at the same conclusion when evaluating unqualified health claims."[3] Although FDA's enforcement of supplement labeling claims has been sporadic, that has not been the case for FTC. Aggressive enforcement against false or misleading advertising has led to large civil fines and disgorgement of unjust profits. In particular, FTC has collected fines and mounted aggressive enforcement of such things as bogus cures, weight loss claims and claims to prevent colds and flu—actions the five trade associations have publicly supported.

In the area of advertising, the industry associations have also pro-actively worked to remind manufacturers and marketers of the restrictions on their advertising and even developed voluntary programs to help police these ads. Four of the five associations have conducted educational programs for their members and the larger industry, to underscore the limits of permissible claims. Three years ago, CRN launched a program with the National Advertising Division (NAD) of the Council of Better Business Bureaus to raise the level of scrutiny of supplement advertising. Through a series of unrestricted grants that total almost $1.5 million funded by CRN, the NAD has been able to add a staff attorney who reviews dietary supplement claims full-time. Challenges can be brought by competitors, consumers, the trade associations or the NAD itself. Claims are evaluated by examining the data submitted by the advertiser itself and written decisions are issued and made public for each case. Since its inception three years ago, the NAD program has issued over 85 opinions that collectively form precedent that guides marketers for future ads. Advertisers who ignore the NAD process or refuse to comply with those decisions do so at their peril: the NAD routinely refers those ads to FTC for follow up and we have been assured those cases get high priority attention for federal investigation.

The Natural Products Foundation (NPF) also maintains a Truth in Advertising program, giving manufacturers the opportunity to pledge to follow FTC's advertising parameters, and notifies manufacturers that it judges to be in violation of the law. If the company does not respond or modify its ads, the NPF notifies FTC and FDA asking that they investigate the charge.

The major media operations that run annual tradeshows for suppliers, manufacturers and retailers also have advertising review programs that screen ads whose claims do not seem to be supported by the evidence. Perhaps more consumer publications should take a cue from these trade journals and institute similar policies not to accept ads containing unsubstantiated or impermissible claims.

So does this mean you will never see a late-night infomercial or a newspaper ad that makes unsupported claims for a dietary supplement? All industries are held hostage to overzealous advertisers. We acknowledge the supplement industry has companies that will push the envelope and even flout the law. Once again, we call upon Congress to provide additional resources to support enforcement activity by both FDA and FTC, along with continued cooperation between these two agencies, to further the critical mission of assuring consumers get accurate information about the dietary supplements they use. New laws that would restrict legitimate commercial speech are neither needed nor appropriate; but rather efforts should be focused on more robust enforcement against the most outlandish of these claims without favoritism against those companies with the deepest pockets.

PRODUCT CLAIMS AT RETAIL

Third, the Committee has exposed some retail salespeople making misguided and impermissible statements for dietary supplements directly to their customers. This is the first time we have heard the audio recordings and we do not know their full extent, or even whether the retailers in the GAO's investigation are aware that they are breaking the law. But as with the previous topics, the Committee should be assured that this kind of behavior is patently illegal and unacceptable. Retailers who make inaccurate or impermissible claims for a dietary supplement have, by their oral comments, misbranded the product at the point of sale under section 403 or the FD&CA, and if the claim is to treat, prevent, cure or mitigate a disease, they have converted the product to an unapproved new drug. These actions also run afoul of the FTC, which has stated that supplement marketers should ensure that *anyone* involved in promoting products is familiar with basic FTC advertising principles. The FTC itself has stated that it "...has taken action not just against supplement manufacturers, but also, in appropriate circumstances, against ad agencies, distributors, retailers, catalog companies, infomercial producers and others involved in deceptive promotions. Therefore, all parties who participate directly or indirectly in the marketing of dietary supplements have an obligation to make sure that claims are presented truthfully and to check the adequacy of the support behind those claims."[4] Furthermore, making a false or misleading statement about a dietary supplement in a consumer transaction violates many states' consumer protection, anti-fraud and unfair competition statutes. In addition, in many states, the licensing requirements for healthcare professionals would make statements about the ability to treat or cure a disease illegal as the unlicensed practice of a medical professional. So there is no question that the legal authority is available to address these marketing practices.

Retailer Education

Whether it is attributable to turnover in the retail sector, new retailers entering the market, or over-enthusiastic testimonials from clerks who are supplement users themselves, the industry recognizes that it is not acceptable for salespeople to make illegal claims to consumers. Here are some of the things we are already doing about it:

- The Natural Products Association has developed a handbook for retailers to assist their retail members with determining their rights and responsibilities under the law. The handbook is clear: You may not diagnose a customer's ailments—that is the practice of medicine. You may not prescribe—suggesting a dietary supplement as an effective treatment or cure of a disease is illegal without a license.
- All the trade associations regularly engage in webinars and symposia to remind their members about what can and cannot be said about supplements. Most of these programs engage officials from FDA and FTC to remind participants of the law, and we are grateful to both agencies for their generous and enthusiastic participation in these industry events. NPA also provides an online quiz for its members "What You Can Tell About the Products You Sell."
- All three major retail vitamin/supplement chains require initial training for all their entry-level employees and provide ongoing continuing education for their retail staff. Other resources include online training, tests for proficiency, monthly newsletters to employees and offsite training sessions that repeatedly remind these employees about the limits on what they can say to consumers.
- Separately, the major direct selling companies who market dietary supplements maintain extensive compliance materials and hold training sessions with their independent distributors to instruct them and reinforce the directive that they may not promote supplement products for diseases or oversell the products' benefits.

However, based on the testimony today, the industry associations recognize that there is more we need to do to give consumers confidence in their supplement purchases. So today, the five associations pledge to the Committee that, either collectively or individually, we will increase our efforts to educate and train retailers who sell dietary supplements and their staffs about what can and cannot legally be said to customers. These efforts may take the form of breakroom posters, brochures that are shipped along with the product, heightened visibility of training events at trade shows or individual follow-up from manufacturers' representatives, but be assured that we take this revelation seriously. We also ask the assistance of FDA and FTC to provide compliance assistance, particularly to small retailers

Consumer Education

But the matter of creating more savvy, more educated consumers is not solely the responsibility of retailers. We also have some simple advice for consumers: the only medical advice consumers should take when it comes to buying supplements is from their healthcare professional—a doctor, a nurse practitioner, a pharmacist, a nurse, a registered dietitian, or a naturopath, for example. Retail professionals—sales clerks, direct sellers, customer service representatives, are there to help customers navigate the retail landscape, to distinguish products, to explain what the products do—but also what the products don't do. Dietary supplements are not intended to treat, prevent or cure disease—and unless a person is working under the guidance of a healthcare professional who is specifically prescribing their care, consumers should not purchase a dietary supplement with that expectation—and a retailer should not sell a dietary supplement with that promise.

Our industry has a responsibility to protect consumers—particularly those who may be more vulnerable to sales pitches—for informing consumers about what supplements reasonably can and cannot do. We echo the well-known adage: if something sounds too good to be true, chances are it is. If, for example, a sales person advises that just by taking a supplement, a person will lose 40 pounds in four weeks, or look 20 years younger, ask for a different salesperson. If a retail clerk tells customers that a supplement product will cure cancer, they should report it to the store's management and walk out of the store immediately. CRN's "Life…supplemented"[5] consumer wellness initiative educates consumers that dietary supplements are an important part of overall wellness, but that they are just one piece of the wellness equation. Consumers shouldn't expect to pop a pill as a magic bullet that will solve their health concerns, but rather should consider incorporating supplements as one of the smart choices they make for healthy living.

Our government has a responsibility too—a responsibility to enforce the law, and a responsibility to educate the public. One of the mandates from DSHEA was to ensure consumers have more information about dietary supplements and FDA and the then newly-formed Office of Dietary Supplements were tasked with this mandate. We would like to see more done in this area and urge the government to find ways to increase public/private partnerships to further educate consumers in this area, so consumers are better able to protect themselves from overzealous or misinformed retailers.

Lastly, despite the issues that have been raised today, we ask the Committee not to lose sight of the important health benefits dietary supplements provide to consumers, specifically to the aging and elderly populations. From the importance of a multivitamin in filling nutritional gaps and helping promote overall good health, to calcium and vitamin D for strong bones; from specialty supplements like omega-3s for supporting heart health to glucosamine and chondroitin for supporting joint health; from botanicals like lutein and bilberry for eye health to saw palmetto for prostate support and to soy and garlic for heart health—dietary supplements are mainstream, affordable options for healthy lifestyles.

The positive health effects of dietary supplements can mean not only a better quality of life for individuals, but also potential positive effects on healthcare cost savings for our country. Studies commissioned by industry and performed by the Lewin Group published between 2003 and 2008 demonstrate significant cost savings in the billions from supplements including calcium, vitamin D, omega-3 fatty acids, lutein, and the multivitamin with folic acid.[6]

CONCLUSION

Dietary supplements offer American consumers, and especially elderly Americans, an effective way to maintain their healthy lifestyles. The vast majority of dietary supplements are safe and beneficial. Those who say all we need to do to protect senior citizens is to change the law, are unfamiliar with the scope of existing law. The framework of the law is substantial—but we need more cops on the beat to make sure it is fully implemented. Give FDA the resources, the support and the clear directive to flex its regulatory muscle.

We also respectfully urge this committee to join Senator Harkin and Senator Hatch in support of their recently introduced bill, the Dietary Supplement Full Implementation and Enforcement Act of 2010; legislation that will provide increased funding for FDA to help ensure the agency has additional resources to implement the current law. This legislation directs the agency to provide annual reports to Congress making itself accountable for enforcing key provisions of the law, just as the industry is responsible for complying with them. Having more laws, without enforcement, only disadvantages the responsible members of industry who do comply with the law because it is the law and because it's the right thing to do for their consumers, and rogue companies will just have more laws to violate. As previous FDA Commissioners have testified to Congress, DSHEA provides more than adequate authority for government while still allowing consumers appropriate access to the products and health information they demand.

Thank you for the opportunity to share our views with the Committee.

This Testimony has been submitted on behalf of the following trade associations:

American Herbal Products Association **(AHPA)** is the national trade association and voice of the herbal products industry. AHPA is comprised of domestic and foreign companies doing business as growers, processors, manufacturers and marketers of herbs and herbal products, including foods, dietary supplements, cosmetics, and nonprescription drugs. Founded in 1982, AHPA's mission is to promote the responsible commerce of herbal products. Website: www.ahpa.org

Consumer Healthcare Products Association **(CHPA)** is the 129-year-old, not-for-profit association representing the makers of over-the-counter medicines and dietary supplements, and the consumers who rely on these healthcare products. Website: www.chpa-info.org.

Council for Responsible Nutrition **(CRN)** represents dietary supplement manufacturers and ingredient suppliers. Its members manufacture popular national brands as well as the store brands marketed by major supermarkets, drug store and discount chains as well as products marketed through natural food stores and direct selling companies. CRN's 70+ manufacturer and supplier members also agree to adhere to voluntary guidelines for formulation, manufacturing, and labeling as well as CRN's Code of Ethics. Website: www.crnusa.org

Natural Products Association **(NPA)**, founded in 1936, is the nation's largest and oldest nonprofit organization dedicated to the natural products industry. The Natural Products Association represents more than 10,000 retailers, manufacturers, wholesalers and distributors of natural products, including foods, dietary supplements, and health/beauty aids. Website: www.npainfo.org

United Natural Products Alliance **(UNPA),** founded in 1991, is an association of dietary supplement and functional food companies that share a commitment to provide consumers with natural health products of superior quality, benefit and reliability. Website: www.unpa.com.

ADDENDUM #1

Healthy Lifestyle Habits of Supplement Users & Non- Users

Below are findings from the 2009 CRN Consumer Survey on Dietary Supplements that examines the healthy habits of supplement users and non-users. The annual survey, which assesses U.S. adults' attitudes and usage of dietary supplements, has been conducted by Ipsos Public Affairs for nearly ten years.

Summary

A larger percentage of supplement users are more likely than non- users to be engaged in the following behaviors: trying to eat a healthy diet, exercising regularly, visiting their doctor regularly, regularly getting a good night's sleep, and maintaining a healthy weight.

Survey question: "I…"	% Agree – Supplement Users	% Agree Don't - Take supplements
Try to eat a balanced diet	88%	76%
Exercise regularly	64%	52%
Visit my doctor regularly	72%	57%
Regularly get a good night's sleep	69%	65%
Maintain a healthy weight	62%	60%

2009 CRN Consumer Survey on Dietary Supplements Methodology: *The 2009 CRN Consumer Survey on Dietary Supplements was conducted August 26 through September 1, 2009 by Ipsos Public Affairs and funded by CRN. The survey was conducted on- line and included a national sample of 2,043 adults aged 18 and older from Ipsos' U.S. on- line panel. The survey has been conducted annually since 2000. Weighting was employed to balance demographics and ensure that the sample's composition reflects that of the U.S. adult population according to Census data and to provide results intended to approximate the sample universe. A survey with an unweighted probability sample of this size would have an estimated margin of error of +/-2.2 percentage points.*

ADDENDUM #2

Life... supplemented™

These are findings from nine healthcare populations surveyed for the 2007- 2009 Healthcare Professionals (HCP) Impact Studies, conducted by the "Life...supplemented" consumer wellness initiative to assess healthcare professionals' personal usage of and recommendations for supplements.

	Population	Use Dietary Supplements (%)	Regular Users (%)	Recommend Dietary Supplements (%)
2007 Oct 2- 11	**Physicians (PCP, Ob/Gyn, Other Specialists)**	**72%**	**51%**	**79%**
	Ob/Gyn (Also included in the results for "Physicians")	**80%**	**56%**	**91%**
	Registered Nurses	**89%**	**59%**	**82%**
2008 Aug 28- Sep 12	**Cardiologists**	**57%**	**37%**	**72%**
	Dermatologists	**75%**	**59%**	**66%**
	Orthopedists	**73%**	**50%**	**91%**
2009 Oct 3- 11	**Nurse Practitioners**	**95%**	**71%**	**96%**
	Registered Dietitians	**96%**	**74%**	**97%**
	Pharmacists	**86%**	**62%**	**93%**

Survey methodologies for all populations can be found at: *http://lifesupplemented.org/supplements/healthcare_professionals_impact_study/methodology.*

End Notes

[1] *See* Addendum #1.
[2] *See* Addendum #2.
[3] http://www.ftc.gov/bcp/edu/pubs/business/adv/bus09.shtm.
[4] http://www.ftc.gov/bcp/edu/pubs/business/adv/bus09.shtm.
[5] www.lifesupplemented.org.
[6] http://www.lewin.com/content/publications/3393.pdf
http://www.lewin.com/content/publications/2833.pdf

In: Dietary Supplements: What Seniors Need to… ISBN: 978-1-61761-285-5
Editors: Thomas H. Felton

Chapter 6

STATEMENT OF JOSHUA M. SHARFSTEIN, M.D., PRINCIPAL DEPUTY COMMISSIONER, U.S. FOOD AND DRUG ADMINISTRATION, DEPT. OF HEALTH AND HUMAN SERVICES, BEFORE THE SENATE SPECIAL COMMITTEE ON AGING, HEARING – "OVERSIGHT OF DIETARY SUPPLEMENTS"

INTRODUCTION

Mr. Chairman and Members of the Committee, I am Dr. Joshua Sharfstein, Principal Deputy Commissioner at the Food and Drug Administration (FDA or the Agency), an agency of the Department of Health and Human Services (HHS).

Thank you for the opportunity to discuss FDA's role in the regulation of dietary supplements, as well as the findings of the study on botanical dietary supplements by the Government Accountability Office (GAO).

Modern FDA oversight of dietary supplements began with the 1994 enactment of the Dietary Supplement Health and Education Act (DSHEA).[1] This regulatory system now includes the following key elements.

1. Prior to its marketing, the manufacturer of a dietary supplement is responsible for ensuring that the supplement is safe;

2. Manufacturers are only permitted to make certain types of claims, and may not make false or misleading claims of any kind;
3. Manufacturers must abide by current Good Manufacturing Practices (cGMPs);
4. Manufacturers must submit to FDA all reports that they receive of serious adverse events associated with a product that it manufactures; and
5. A manufacturer must submit a notification to FDA before it markets a dietary supplement containing a "New Dietary Ingredient."

1. Responsibility for Safety

FDA does not approve dietary supplements before they reach the consumer. Rather, manufacturers of dietary supplements are responsible for ensuring that the supplement is safe before marketing.

In the case of a new dietary ingredient (described further below), a premarket submission of data and information regarding the safety of the product is required by law. Otherwise, a firm does not have to provide FDA with the evidence on safety before it markets its products.

Generally, manufacturers register their facilities but do not register their products with FDA.

2. Claims

Under the law, claims that are allowed to be used on food and dietary supplement labels fall into three categories: health claims, nutrient content claims, and structure/function claims. Disease-related claims are generally not permitted for dietary supplements.

Health Claims

Health claims describe a relationship between a dietary supplement ingredient and a reduction in the risk of a disease or health-related condition.[2] FDA's oversight has three components:

First, under the Nutrition Labeling and Education Act of 1990 (NLEA), FDA issues regulations authorizing health claims for dietary supplements after FDA's review of the scientific evidence submitted in health claim petitions.

Second, the 1997 Food and Drug Administration Modernization Act authorizes health claims based on an authoritative statement of a scientific body of the U.S. government with official responsibility for public health protection or research directly related to human nutrition, or the National Academy of Sciences. Such claims may be used after submission of a health claim notification to FDA.

Third, FDA permits some health claims that are not authorized by regulation but are supported by credible evidence and accompanied by a non-misleading disclaimer. Such claims are referred to as "qualified health claims." For example: "One small study suggests that chromium picolinate may reduce the risk of insulin resistance, and therefore possibly may reduce the risk of type 2 diabetes. FDA concludes, however, that the existence of such a relationship between chromium picolinate and either insulin resistance or type 2 diabetes is highly uncertain."

Nutrient Content Claims

NLEA permits the use of claims that characterize the level of a nutrient in a food or dietary supplement made in accordance with FDA regulations.

Nutrient content claims describe the level of a nutrient or dietary substance in the product, using terms such as free, high, and low, or they compare the level of a nutrient in a food to that of another food, using terms such as more, reduced, and "lite." Most nutrient content claim regulations apply only to those nutrients or dietary substances that have an established daily value.

The regulations that govern the use of nutrient content claims help ensure that descriptive terms, such as high or low, are used consistently for all types of food products (including dietary supplements) and are meaningful to consumers.

Percentage claims for dietary supplements are another category of nutrient content claims. These claims are used to describe a level of a dietary ingredient for which there is no established Daily Value. Examples include simple percentage statements such as "40% omega-3 fatty acids, 10 mg per capsule," and comparative percentage claims, e.g., "twice the omega-3 fatty acids per capsule (80 mg) as in 100 mg of menhaden oil (40 mg)."

Structure/Function Claims

DSHEA established special regulatory procedures for structure/function claims for dietary supplement labels.

Structure/function claims describe the role of a nutrient or dietary ingredient intended to affect normal structure or function in humans. Examples of these claims include "calcium builds strong bones" and "fiber maintains bowel regularity."

Structure/function claims may also describe a benefit related to a nutrient deficiency disease, as long as the statement also tells how widespread such a disease is in the United States.

Manufacturers are responsible for ensuring the accuracy and truthfulness of these claims. Such claims are not pre-approved by FDA. If a dietary supplement label includes a structure/function claim, Section 403(r)(6) of the Act and its implementing regulation at 21 *Code of Federal Regulations* 101.93(b) require that the label state in a "disclaimer" that FDA has not evaluated the claim. The disclaimer must also state that the dietary supplement product is not intended to "diagnose, treat, cure or prevent any disease," because only a drug can legally make such a claim under the FD&C Act.

Dietary supplement manufacturers that make structure/function claims on labels or in labeling must submit a notification to FDA no later than 30 days after marketing the dietary supplement that includes the text of the claim. FDA has provided industry with guidance on these requirements.

Generally Not Permitted: Disease-Related Claims

Dietary supplements are generally not permitted to claim to act as a treatment, prevention or cure for a disease or condition. Such claims are generally reserved for drugs and require pre-approval by FDA. The only exception is that supplements may claim a benefit related to a classical nutrient deficiency disease, provided that they also disclose the prevalence of the disease in the United States.

3. Current Good Manufacturing Practices

DSHEA provides express authority for regulations establishing cGMP requirements for dietary supplements.

In June 2007, FDA promulgated a final rule establishing these cGMPs, under which manufacturers are required to evaluate the identity, purity, quality, strength, and composition of dietary supplements. The final rule aims to avoid wrong ingredients; too much or too little of a dietary ingredient; improper packaging; improper labeling; or contamination problems due to natural toxins, bacteria, pesticides, glass, lead, or other substances.

To limit any disruption for dietary supplements produced by small businesses, the rule has a three-year phase-in for small businesses. The largest firms, with more than 500 employees, were subject to compliance beginning in June 2008; mid-size firms in June 2009; the smallest firms, with fewer than 20 employees, will be expected to be in compliance with the cGMPs this June.

Since the final rule was released, FDA has trained both industry stakeholders and FDA staff on the requirements of the regulations. Violations of the regulations are violations of the law and can lead to both civil and criminal penalties.

Since the rule went into effect in June 2008, we have conducted approximately 55 inspections for compliance with the new regulations. The majority of facilities have been found to be in substantial compliance.

4. Adverse Event Reporting

As of December 2007, manufacturers, packers, and distributors of dietary supplements must forward to FDA any reports they receive of serious adverse events associated with the use of those products. These firms must also keep records about each adverse event report they receive and provide FDA with access to these records during inspections.

The Agency evaluates the serious adverse event reports, and any other adverse event information reported voluntarily by healthcare providers, firms, or consumers, to identify signals that a product may present safety risks to consumers. FDA received 1,107 serious adverse event reports in 2008 and 1,275 reports in 2009.

5. New Dietary Ingredients

The FD&C Act requires that manufacturers and distributors who wish to market dietary supplements that contain "new dietary ingredients" (NDIs) provide FDA with information regarding the safety of such a dietary supplement before marketing.[3] Ingredients marketed in food in the United States prior to passage of DHSEA are not "new dietary ingredients" and are thus grandfathered out of this requirement, as are many ingredients introduced into the food supply after 1994, such as those introduced for use in conventional foods.

There is no authoritative list of ingredients that were marketed prior to 1994, which creates a significant challenge to FDA in enforcing this provision of the Act.

FDA is developing a guidance document on what should be considered in determining the status of an ingredient as an NDI, what information should be submitted about a dietary supplement containing the NDI, and how a reasonable expectation of safety of the NDI should be established. We expect this guidance document to be ready by the end of this year.

FDA's Enforcement Priorities

FDA monitors products on the market for safety by reviewing adverse event reports, obtaining information from inspections of dietary supplement manufacturers and distributors, reviewing consumer and trade complaints, performing laboratory analyses of product samples, and monitoring retail outlets, including the Internet.

The Agency also monitors product information, such as labeling, package inserts, and accompanying literature, for potentially false or misleading claims. Our regulatory partners at the Federal Trade Commission (FTC) have authority over dietary supplement advertising.

Currently, the Agency focuses enforcement actions related to dietary supplements on three areas that pose the greatest risk to public health.

Adulteration with Drug Substances

Products that are marketed as dietary supplements but contain active ingredients in FDA-approved drugs, analogs of approved drugs, and other compounds that do not qualify as dietary ingredients, present an emerging and expanding challenge.

FDA has found that certain products in the following categories have been illegally represented as dietary supplements: sexual enhancement or erectile dysfunction, weight loss, cholesterol reduction, and body building products. These products have been found to be intended for use as drugs and to contain active prescription pharmaceutical ingredients including PDE-5 Inhibitors (e.g., sildenafil or Viagra), controlled substances for obesity (e.g., sibutramine or Meridia), lovastatin, and synthetic steroids or steroid-like substances.

These products are often sold with misleading labeling and are frequently manufactured without quality controls.

A challenge for enforcement is that some of these chemicals can be difficult to detect. Nonetheless, in the last two years:

FDA has participated in the voluntary recall of dozens upon dozens of tainted supplement products, including:

- More than 50 sexual enhancement supplements, including a rare "FDA-requested" recall;
- More than 40 weight loss supplements; and
- More than 80 body building supplements by two distributors alone.

The Agency has issued multiple consumer alerts and press announcements to warn consumers about hazardous products. These include:

- Four warnings about individual firms marketing sexual enhancement products in cases in which FDA was unable to secure acknowledgement of an appropriate action to remove the products from commerce;
- Multiple consumer alerts concerning more than 70 tainted weight loss supplements; and
- A public health advisory issued about body building products that are represented as containing steroids or steroid-like substances.

We have has participated in seizures and criminal prosecutions to disrupt the distribution of illegal products, including:

- Two civil seizures of illegal sexual enhancement supplements in 2009;
- Two individuals arrested for illegally trafficking weight loss "supplements"; and
- Multiple search warrant affidavits served on firms marketing body building products that are represented as containing steroids or steroid-like substances, with one manufacturer pleading guilty to selling the illegal products.

Illegal Claims

Dietary supplements with unsubstantiated and illegal claims may encourage consumers to self-treat for a serious disease without the benefit of a medical diagnosis or treatment. FDA conducts enforcement activities against supplements that make these types of claims.

For example, on March 31, 2010, the United States Marshal for the Western District of Wisconsin seized a range of dietary supplements and other products from a firm that was promoting the products for unapproved uses. The firm promoted its bee-derived products to treat, cure or prevent diseases and conditions such as cancer, asthma, arthritis and hypertension.

In response to the H1N1 flu crisis of 2009, FDA launched an initiative to address the numerous fraudulent products that were promoted to treat, prevent, or cure H1N1 flu. The Agency targeted products that were promoted on the Internet and issued Warning Letters to the owners of the websites. Approximately 70 products were supplements. In addition to the Warning Letters issued solely by FDA, FDA and FTC issued one joint letter to a supplement firm. This was the first joint FDA/FTC advisory letter.

Unsafe Ingredients

A dietary supplement is adulterated, and subject to enforcement action, "if it bears or contains any poisonous or deleterious substance which may render it injurious to health" or if it presents a "significant or unreasonable" risk to consumers. DSHEA allows the HHS Secretary to ban a dietary supplement if she finds it to be an "imminent hazard."

Under the current regulatory framework, FDA looks for such problems after marketing through reviewing the medical literature and analyzing adverse event reports. Because many products have multiple ingredients, it is challenging to identify causal connections between specific ingredients and adverse effects.

In 2009, FDA became aware of serious problems associated with a supplement product called Hydroxycut. Many of the reports advised of serious liver injuries, including liver damage that required transplants. After discussion with the Agency, the manufacturer voluntarily recalled Hydroxycut and subsequently reformulated the products.

GAO Study

Since October 2009, GAO has been conducting an investigation, at the request of this Committee, into the manufacturing and marketing of dietary supplements, particularly botanical products. GAO has discussed its findings with FDA and we have provided GAO with our comments.

During their inquiry into the marketing of herbal dietary supplements, GAO investigators found a number of claims that appear to cause the products to be illegal. In general, these claims promised cures for diseases and conditions. When FDA identifies such claims in the labeling of products on the market, the Agency takes action.

GAO also analyzed 40 dietary supplements for heavy metal contaminants. All of the products were found to contain trace amounts of lead, cadmium, arsenic and mercury. Given the expected generally small consumption of the supplements, we do not believe these levels represent a significant risk to health. For example, the cadmium levels reached to about 1.4 μg/day (micrograms per day). This compares to FDA's tolerable daily intake level of 60 μg/day.

The lead levels reached to 1.9 μg/day, which is about a third of FDA's tolerable daily intake. While this is a not a dangerous level, it is a significant fraction of daily intake. It is possible that preventive standards of the type authorized by pending food safety legislation could help FDA reduce lead levels in dietary supplements as much as feasible.

Recently, FDA and the New York City Health Department identified lead in a dietary supplement at a level of 1,100 parts per million (ppm) -- more than 10,000 times higher than FDA's maximum recommended level for lead in certain candies. We immediately notified the public of a potential risk and inspected the facility, and the manufacturer recalled the supplement.

GAO also analyzed supplements for pesticide residues. The 41 residues listed in Appendix IV of GAO's statement of facts fall into four groups.

- Seven residues were found at levels within the Environmental Protection Agency (EPA) tolerances for dietary supplements. For example, two samples of ginseng had residues of metalaxyl at .01 and .03 parts per billion (ppb), while the tolerance level for metalaxyl in ginseng is set by EPA at 3.0 ppb.
- Thirty-one (31) residues were at levels within tolerances used for fruits and vegetables, but there are no tolerances in the law for dietary supplements. For example, the pesticide chlorpyrifos has no set tolerance level for residue in Echinacea, where it was found at a level of .01 ppm. However, residue levels for chlorpyrifos have been set for celery at 15 ppm and for tomatoes at 5 ppm.
- One residue found was a low level of carbofuran, a pesticide that had its tolerances canceled by EPA in 2009.
- Two residues were low levels of pesticides that were either never approved for use in the United States (tolclofos-methyl) or had their use banned in the United States over 40 years ago (hexachlorobenzene, or HCB). These findings are within or very close to the allowable residue levels set by the European Union.

FDA presently analyzes close to two hundred herbal and botanical products annually in our pesticide monitoring program. When violations are found on imported dietary supplements, products are typically put on Detention Without Physical Examination, under which entries of such products are refused admission into United States commerce unless acceptable evidence is provided to the Agency demonstrating compliance with applicable requirements. Likewise, when violations are found on domestically-produced dietary supplements, the product is removed from commerce.

CONCLUSION

Thank you for the opportunity to discuss FDA's activities with regard to dietary supplements. FDA looks forward to working with Congress on this important public health issue.

I look forward to your questions.

End Notes

[1] The Federal Food, Drug, and Cosmetic Act (FD&C Act or the Act) defines a "dietary ingredient" as a vitamin, a mineral, an amino acid, an herb or other botanical, or a dietary substance for use by man to supplement the diet by increasing the total dietary intake, or a concentrate, metabolite, constituent, extract, or combination of any of the above dietary ingredients. Dietary supplements must be intended for ingestion and may be found in many forms such as tablets, capsules, powder, liquids, softgels, or gelcaps. Importantly, under the Act, a dietary supplement may not contain an article approved as a new drug or an article authorized for investigation as a new drug for which substantial clinical investigations have been instituted and made public, unless the article was first marketed as a dietary supplement or conventional food. DSHEA defines the term "dietary supplement" as a product that, among other things, is not represented for use as a conventional food or sole item in a meal or diet; is intended to supplement the diet; and contains at least one or more dietary ingredients.

[2] A health claim by definition has two essential components: 1) a substance (the dietary supplement or ingredient) and 2) a characterization of its relationship to a disease or health-related condition.

[3] A "new dietary ingredient" (NDI) is a dietary ingredient not marketed in the United States in a dietary supplement before October 15, 1994. The notification must include information on the basis on which the manufacturer or distributor concluded that a dietary supplement containing a new dietary ingredient will reasonably be expected to be safe. For 75 days after the filing date, the notifier may not market the dietary supplement that contains the NDI. During the 75-day period, FDA may ask the notifier for more information, which may reset the review clock. If FDA has no objection, it can acknowledge the notification but does not issue an "approval" regulation as it does for drugs or food additives.

In: Dietary Supplements: What Seniors Need to… ISBN: 978-1-61761-285-5
Editors: Thomas H. Felton

Chapter 7

AGE PAGE: DIETARY SUPPLEMENTS

National Institute on Aging

Bill's retired and lives alone. Often he's just not hungry or is too tired to fix a whole meal. Does he need a multivitamin, or should he take one of those dietary supplements he sees in ads everywhere? Bill wonders if they work—will one help keep his joints healthy or another give him more energy? And, are they safe?

WHAT IS A DIETARY SUPPLEMENT?

Dietary supplements are substances you might use to add nutrients to your diet or to lower your risk of health problems, like osteoporosis or arthritis. Dietary supplements come in the form of pills, capsules, powders, gel tabs, extracts, or liquids. They might contain vitamins, minerals, fiber, amino acids, herbs or other plants, or enzymes. Sometimes, the ingredients in dietary supplements are added to foods, including drinks. A doctor's prescription is not needed to buy dietary supplements.

Should I Take a Dietary Supplement?

Do you need one? Maybe you do, but usually not. Ask yourself why you think you might want to take a dietary supplement. Are you concerned about getting enough nutrients? Is a friend, a neighbor, or someone on a commercial suggesting you take one? Some ads for dietary supplements in magazines or on TV seem to promise that these supplements will make you feel better, keep you from getting sick, or even help you live longer. Sometimes, there is little, if any, good scientific research supporting these claims. Some dietary supplements will give you nutrients that might be missing from your daily diet. But eating healthy foods is the best way to get the nutrients you need. Others may cost a lot or might not benefit you the way you would like. Some supplements can change how medicines you may already be taking will work. You should talk to your doctor or a registered dietitian for advice.

What If I'm over 50?

People over 50 need more of some vitamins and minerals than younger adults do. Your doctor or a dietitian can tell you whether you need to change your diet or take vitamins or minerals to get enough of these:

- **Vitamin B_{12}**. Vitamin B_{12} helps keep your red blood cells and nerves healthy. As people grow older, some have trouble absorbing vitamin B_{12} naturally found in food. Instead, they can choose foods, like fortified cereals, that have this vitamin added or use a B_{12} supplement.
- **Calcium**. Calcium works with vitamin D to keep bones strong at all ages. Bone loss can lead to fractures in both older women and men. Calcium is found in milk and milk products (fat-free or low-fat is best), canned fish with soft bones, dark-green leafy vegetables like spinach, and foods with calcium added.
- **Vitamin D**. Some people's bodies make enough vitamin D if they are in the sun for 10 to 15 minutes at least twice a week. But, if you are older, you may not be able to get enough vitamin D that way. Try adding vitamin D-fortified milk and milk products, vitamin D-fortified cereals, and fatty fish to your diet, and/or use a vitamin D supplement.

- **Vitamin B_6**. This vitamin is needed to form red blood cells. It is found in potatoes, bananas, chicken breasts, and fortified cereals.

DIFFERENT VITAMIN AND MINERAL RECOMMENDATIONS FOR PEOPLE OVER 50

The National Academy of Sciences recommends how much of each vitamin and mineral men and women of different ages need. Sometimes, the Academy also tells us how much of a vitamin or mineral is too much.

Vitamin B_{12}—2.4 mcg (micrograms) each day (if you are taking medicine for acid reflux, you might need a different form, which your health care provider can give you)

Calcium—1200 mg (milligrams), but not more than 2500 mg a day

Vitamin D—400 IU (International Units) for people age 51 to 70 and 600 IU for those over 70, but not more than 2000 IU each day

Vitamin B_6—1.7 mg for men and 1.5 mg for women each day

When thinking about whether you need more of a vitamin or mineral, think about how much of each nutrient you get from food and drinks, as well as from any supplements you take. Check with a doctor or dietitian to learn whether you need to supplement your diet.

WHAT ARE ANTIOXIDANTS?

You might hear about *antioxidants* in the news. These are natural substances found in food that might help protect you from some diseases. Here are some common sources of antioxidants that you should be sure to include in your diet:

- *beta-carotene*—fruits and vegetables that are either dark green or dark orange
- *selenium*—seafood, liver, meat, and grains
- *vitamin C*—citrus fruits, peppers, tomatoes, and berries

- *vitamin E*—wheat germ, nuts, sesame seeds, and canola, olive, and peanut oils

Right now, research results suggest that large doses of supplements with antioxidants will not prevent chronic diseases such as heart disease or diabetes. In fact, some studies have shown that taking large doses of some antioxidants could be harmful. Again, it is best to check with your doctor before taking a dietary supplement.

What about Herbal Supplements?

Herbal supplements are dietary supplements that come from plants. A few that you may have heard of are gingko biloba, ginseng, echinacea, and black cohosh. Researchers are looking at using herbal supplements to prevent or treat some health problems. It's too soon to know if herbal supplements are both safe and useful. But, studies of some have not shown benefits.

Are Dietary Supplements Safe?

Scientists are still working to answer this question. The U.S. Food and Drug Administration (FDA) checks prescription medicines, such as antibiotics or blood pressure medicines, to make sure they are safe and do what they promise. The same is true for over-the-counter drugs like pain and cold medicines.

But the FDA does not consider dietary supplements to be medicines. The FDA does not watch over dietary supplements in the same way it does prescription medicines. The Federal Government does not regularly test what is in dietary supplements. So, just because you see a dietary supplement on a store shelf does not mean it is safe or that it even does what the label says it will or contains what the label says it contains.

If the FDA receives reports of possible problems with a supplement, it will issue warnings about products that are clearly unsafe. The FDA may also take these supplements off the market. The Federal Trade Commission looks into reports of ads that might misrepresent what dietary supplements do.

A few private groups, such as the U.S. Pharmacopeia (USP), NSF International, ConsumerLab.com, and the Natural Products Association

(NPA), have their own "seals of approval" for dietary supplements. To get such a seal, products must be made by following good manufacturing procedures, must contain what is listed on the label, and must not have harmful levels of things that don't belong there, like lead.

WHAT'S BEST FOR ME?

If you are thinking about using dietary supplements:

- **Learn.** Find out as much as you can about any dietary supplement you might take. Talk to your doctor, your pharmacist, or a registered dietitian. A supplement that seemed to help your neighbor might not work for you. If you are reading fact sheets or checking websites, be aware of the source of the information. Could the writer or group profit from the sale of a particular supplement? For more information from the National Institute on Aging about choosing reliable health information websites, see *For More Information.*
- **Remember.** Just because something is said to be "natural" doesn't also mean it is either safe or good for you. It could have side effects. It might make a medicine your doctor prescribed for you either weaker or stronger.
- **Tell your doctor.** He or she needs to know if you decide to go ahead and use a dietary supplement. Do not diagnose or treat your health condition without first checking with your doctor.
- **Buy wisely.** Choose brands that your doctor, dietitian, or pharmacist says are trustworthy. Don't buy dietary supplements with ingredients you don't need. Don't assume that more of something that might be good for you is even better for you.
- **Check the science.** Make sure any claim made about a dietary supplement is based on scientific proof. The company making the dietary supplement should be able to send you information on the safety and/or effectiveness of the ingredients in a product, which you can then discuss with your doctor. Remember that if something sounds too good to be true, it probably is.

What Can I Do to Stay Healthy?

Here's what one active older person does:

When she turned 60, Pearl decided she wanted to stay healthy and active as long as possible. She was careful about what she ate. She became more physically active. Now she takes a long, brisk walk 3 or 4 times a week. In bad weather, she joins the mall walkers at the local shopping mall. When it's nice outside, Pearl works in her garden. When she was younger, Pearl stopped smoking and started using a seatbelt. She's even learning how to use a computer to find healthy recipes. Last month, she danced at her granddaughter's wedding. Pearl is 84 years old.

Try following Pearl's example—stick to a healthy diet, be physically active, keep your mind active, don't smoke, see your doctor regularly, and, in most cases, only use dietary supplements suggested by your doctor or pharmacist.

For More Information

Here are some helpful resources:

Department of Agriculture
Food and Nutrition Information Center
National Agricultural Library
10301 Baltimore Avenue, Room 105
Beltsville, MD 20705-2351
301-504-5414
www.nal.usda.gov/fnic

Federal Trade Commission
600 Pennsylvania Avenue, NW
Washington, DC 20580
877-382-4357 (toll-free)
202-326-2222
www.ftc.gov/healthclaims

Food and Drug Administration
Center for Food Safety and
Applied Nutrition
5100 Paint Branch Parkway HFS-555
College Park, MD 20740-3835
888-723-3366 (toll-free)
www.cfsan.fda.gov

National Center for Complementary and Alternative Medicine
NCCAM Clearinghouse
Box 7923
Gaithersburg, MD 20898
888-644-6226 (toll-free)
866-464-3615 (TTY/toll-free)
www.nccam.nih.gov

National Library of Medicine MedlinePlus
www.medlineplus.gov

Office of Dietary Supplements
6100 Executive Boulevard
Room 3B01, MSC 7517
Bethesda, MD 20892-7517
301-435-2920
www.ods.od.nih.gov
The Federal Government has several other websites with information on nutrition, including:
www.nutrition.gov—learn more about healthy eating, food shopping, assistance programs, and nutritionrelated health subjects.
www.mypyramid.gov—information about the *Dietary Guidelines for Americans.*

For information on exercise, nutrition, and health quackery and other resources on health and aging, contact:

National Institute on Aging Information Center
P.O. Box 8057
Gaithersburg, MD 20898-8057
800-222-2225 (toll-free)
800-222-4225 (TTY/toll-free)

www.nia.nih.gov
www.nia.nih.gov/Espanol

To sign up for regular email alerts about new publications and other information from the NIA, go to www.nia.nih.gov/HealthInformation.

Visit NIHSeniorHealth (www.nihseniorhealth.gov), a seniorfriendly website from the National Institute on Aging and National Library of Medicine. This website has health information for older adults. Special features make it simple to use. For example, you can click on a button to have the text read out loud or to make the type larger.

In: Dietary Supplements: What Seniors Need to... ISBN: 978-1-61761-285-5
Editors: Thomas H. Felton

Chapter 8

FDA 101: DIETARY SUPPLEMENTS

Consumer Health Information

The law defines dietary supplements in part as products taken by mouth that contain a "dietary ingredient." Dietary ingredients include vitamins, minerals, amino acids, and herbs or botanicals, as well as other substances that can be used to supplement the diet.

Dietary supplements come in many forms, including tablets, capsules, powders, energy bars, and liquids. These products are available in stores throughout the United States, as well as on the Internet. They are labeled as dietary supplements and include among others

- vitamin and mineral products
- "botanical" or herbal products—These come in many forms and may include plant materials, algae, macroscopic fungi, or a combination of these materials.
- amino acid products—Amino acids are known as the building blocks of proteins and play a role in metabolism.
- enzyme supplements—Enzymes are complex proteins that speed up biochemical reactions.

People use dietary supplements for a wide assortment of reasons. Some seek to compensate for diets, medical conditions, or eating habits that limit the intake of essential vitamins and nutrients. Other people look to them to boost energy or to get a good night's sleep. Postmenopausal women consider using them to counter a sudden drop in estrogen levels.

FDA suggests that you consult with a health care professional before using any dietary supplement.

Using supplements improperly can be harmful. Taking a combination of supplements, using these products together with medicine, or substituting them in place of prescribed medicines could lead to harmful, even life-threatening, results.

Talk with a Health Care Professional

The Food and Drug Administration (FDA) suggests that you consult with a health care professional before using any dietary supplement. Many supplements contain ingredients that have strong biological effects, and such products may not be safe in all people.

If you have certain health conditions and take these products, you may be putting yourself at risk. Your health care professional can discuss with you whether it is safe for you to take a particular product and whether the product is appropriate for your needs. Here is some general advice:

- **Dietary supplements are not intended to treat, diagnose, cure, or alleviate the effects of diseases.** They cannot completely prevent diseases, as some vaccines can. However, some supplements are useful in reducing the risk of certain diseases and are authorized to make label claims about these uses. For example, folic acid supplements may make a claim about reducing the risk of birth defects of the brain and spinal cord.
- **Using supplements improperly can be harmful.** Taking a combination of supplements, using these products together with medicine, or substituting them in place of prescribed medicines could lead to harmful, even life-threatening, results.
- **Some supplements can have unwanted effects before, during, or after surgery.** For example, bleeding is a potential side effect risk of garlic, ginkgo biloba, ginseng, and Vitamin E. In addition, kava and valerian act as sedatives and can increase the effects of anesthetics

and other medications used during surgery. Before surgery, you should inform your health care professional about all the supplements you use.

How Are Supplements Regulated?

You should know the following if you are considering using a dietary supplement.

- Federal law requires that every dietary supplement be labeled as such, either with the term "dietary supplement" or with a term that substitutes a description of the product's dietary ingredient(s) for the word "dietary" (e.g., "herbal supplement" or "calcium supplement").
- Federal law does not require dietary supplements to be proven safe to FDA's satisfaction before they are marketed.
- For most claims made in the labeling of dietary supplements, the law does not require the manufacturer or seller to prove to FDA's satisfaction that the claim is accurate or truthful before it appears on the product.
- In general, FDA's role with a dietary supplement product begins after the product enters the marketplace. That is usually the agency's first opportunity to take action against a product that presents a significant or unreasonable risk of illness or injury, or that is otherwise adulterated or misbranded.
- Dietary supplement advertising, including ads broadcast on radio and television, falls under the jurisdiction of the Federal Trade Commission.
- Once a dietary supplement is on the market, FDA has certain safety monitoring responsibilities. These include monitoring mandatory reporting of serious adverse events by dietary supplement firms and voluntary adverse event reporting by consumers and health care professionals. As its resources permit, FDA also reviews product labels and other product information, such as package inserts, accompanying literature, and Internet promotion.
- Dietary supplement firms must report to FDA any serious adverse events that are reported to them by consumers or health care professionals.

- Dietary supplement manufacturers do not have to get the agency's approval before producing or selling these products.
- It is not legal to market a dietary supplement product as a treatment or cure for a specific disease, or to alleviate the symptoms of a disease.
- There are limitations to FDA oversight of claims in dietary supplement labeling. For example, FDA reviews substantiation for claims as resources permit.

Are Supplements Safe?

Many dietary supplements have clean safety histories. For example, millions of Americans responsibly consume multi-vitamins and experience no ill effects.

Some dietary supplements have been shown to be beneficial for certain health conditions. For example, the use of folic acid supplements by women of childbearing age who may become pregnant reduces the risk of some birth defects.

Another example is the crystalline form of vitamin B12, which is beneficial in people over age 50 who often have a reduced ability to absorb naturally occurring vitamin B12. But further study is needed for some other dietary supplements.

Some ingredients and products can be harmful when consumed in high amounts, when taken for a long time, or when used in combination with certain other drugs, substances, or foods.

Some supplements have had to be recalled because of proven or potential harmful effects. Reasons for these recalls include

- microbiological, pesticide, and heavy metal contamination
- absence of a dietary ingredient claimed to be in the product
- the presence of more or less than the amount of the dietary ingredient claimed on the label

In addition, unscrupulous manufacturers have tried to sell bogus products that should not be on the market at all.

Before taking a dietary supplement, make sure that the supplement is safe for you and appropriate for the intended purpose.

BE A SAFE AND INFORMED CONSUMER

- Let your health care professional advise you on sorting reliable information from questionable information.
- Contact the manufacturer for information about the product you intend to use.
- Be aware that some supplement ingredients, including nutrients and plant components, can be toxic. Also, some ingredients and products can be harmful when consumed in high amounts, when taken for a long time, or when used in combination with certain other drugs, substances, or foods.
- Do not self-diagnose any health condition. Work with health care professionals to determine how best to achieve optimal health.
- Do not substitute a dietary supplement for a prescription medicine or therapy, or for the variety of foods important to a healthful diet.
- Do not assume that the term "natural" in relation to a product ensures that the product is wholesome or safe.
- Be wary of hype and headlines. Sound health advice is generally based upon research over time, not a single study.
- Learn to spot false claims. If something sounds too good to be true, it probably is.

REPORT PROBLEMS

Adverse effects with dietary supplements should be reported to FDA as soon as possible. If you experience such an adverse effect, contact or see your health care professional immediately. Both of you are then encouraged to report this problem to FDA. For information on how to do this, go to www.cfsan.fda.gov/~dms/ds-rept.html.

Adverse effects can also be reported to the product's manufacturer or distributor through the address or phone number listed on the product's label. Dietary supplement firms are required to forward reports they receive about serious adverse effects to FDA within 15 days.

For a general, nonserious complaint or concern about dietary supplements, contact your local FDA District Office (www.cfsan.fda.gov/~dms/district.html).

This article appears on FDA's Consumer Health Information Web page (www.fda.gov/consumer), which features the latest updates on FDA-regulated products. Sign up for free e-mail subscriptions at *www.fda.gov/consumer/cons* umerenews.html.

For More Information

Protect Your Health
Joint FDA/WebMD resource
www.webmd.com/fda

Fortify Your Knowledge About
Vitamins
www.fda.gov/consumer/updates/vitamins111907.html

Tips for the Savvy Supplement User:
Making Informed Decisions
www.fda.gov/fdac/features/2002/202_supp.html

Overview of Dietary Supplements
www.cfsan.fda.gov/~dms/ds-oview.html#what

Food Labeling and Nutrition
www.cfsan.fda.gov/label.html

Final Rule Promotes Safe Use of Dietary Supplements
www.fda.gov/consumer/updates/dietarysupps062207.html

In: Dietary Supplements: What Seniors Need to... ISBN: 978-1-61761-285-5
Editors: Thomas H. Felton

Chapter 9

USING DIETARY SUPPLEMENTS WISELY

United States Department of Health and Human Services

Many people take dietary supplements in an effort to be well and stay healthy. With so many dietary supplements available and so many claims made about their health benefits, how can a consumer decide what's safe and effective? This fact sheet provides a general overview of dietary supplements, discusses safety considerations, and suggests sources for additional information.

KEY POINTS

- Federal regulations for dietary supplements are very different from those for prescription and over-the-counter drugs. For example, a dietary supplement manufacturer does not have to prove a product's safety and effectiveness before it is marketed.
- If you are thinking about using a dietary supplement, first get information on it from reliable sources. Keep in mind that dietary supplements may interact with medications or other dietary supplements and may contain ingredients not listed on the label.
- Tell your health care providers about any complementary and alternative practices you use, including dietary supplements. Give

them a full picture of what you do to manage your health. This will help ensure coordinated and safe care.

About Dietary Supplements

Dietary supplements were defined in a law passed by Congress in 1994 called the Dietary Supplement Health and Education Act (DSHEA). According to DSHEA, a dietary supplement is a product that:

- Is intended to supplement the diet
- Contains one or more dietary ingredients (including vitamins, minerals, herbs or other botanicals, amino acids, and certain other substances) or their constituents
- Is intended to be taken by mouth, in forms such as tablet, capsule, powder, softgel, gelcap, or liquid
- Is labeled as being a dietary supplement.

Herbal supplements are one type of dietary supplement. An herb is a plant or plant part (such as leaves, flowers, or seeds) that is used for its flavor, scent, and/or therapeutic properties. "Botanical" is often used as a synonym for "herb." An herbal supplement may contain a single herb or mixtures of herbs.

Research has shown that some uses of dietary supplements are effective in preventing or treating diseases. For example, scientists have found that folic acid (a vitamin) prevents certain birth defects, and a regimen of vitamins and zinc can slow the progression of the age-related eye disease macular degeneration. Also, calcium and vitamin D supplements can be helpful in preventing and treating bone loss and osteoporosis (thinning of bone tissue).

Research has also produced some promising results suggesting that other dietary supplements may be helpful for other health conditions (e.g., omega-3 fatty acids for coronary disease), but in most cases, additional research is needed before firm conclusions can be drawn.

Dietary Supplement Use in the United States

A national survey conducted in 2007 found that 17.7 percent of American adults had used "natural products" (i.e., dietary supplements other than vitamins and minerals) in the past 12 months. The most popular products used by adults for health reasons in the past 30 days were fish oil/omega 3/DHA (37.4 percent), glucosamine (19.9 percent), echinacea (19.8 percent), flaxseed oil or pills (15.9 percent), and ginseng (14.1 percent). In another, earlier national survey covering all types of dietary supplements, approximately 52 percent of adult respondents said they had used some type of supplement in the last 30 days; the most commonly reported were multivitamins/multiminerals (35 percent), vitamins E and C (12-13 percent), calcium (10 percent), and B-complex vitamins (5 percent).

FEDERAL REGULATION OF DIETARY SUPPLEMENTS

The Federal Government regulates dietary supplements through the U.S. Food and Drug Administration (FDA). The regulations for dietary supplements are not the same as those for prescription or over-the-counter drugs. In general, the regulations for dietary supplements are less strict.

- A manufacturer does not have to prove the safety and effectiveness of a dietary supplement before it is marketed. A manufacturer is permitted to say that a dietary supplement addresses a nutrient deficiency, supports health, or is linked to a particular body function (e.g., immunity), if there is research to support the claim. Such a claim must be followed by the words "This statement has not been evaluated by the U.S. Food and Drug Administration (FDA). This product is not intended to diagnose, treat, cure, or prevent any disease."
- Manufacturers are expected to follow certain "good manufacturing practices" (GMPs) to ensure that dietary supplements are processed consistently and meet quality standards. Requirements for GMPs went into effect in 2008 for large manufacturers and are being phased in for small manufacturers through 2010.
- Once a dietary supplement is on the market, the FDA monitors safety. If it finds a product to be unsafe, it can take action against the manufacturer and/or distributor, and may issue a warning or require that the product be removed from the marketplace.

Also, once a dietary supplement is on the market, the FDA monitors product information, such as label claims and package inserts. The Federal

Trade Commission (FTC) is responsible for regulating product advertising; it requires that all information be truthful and not misleading.

The Federal Government has taken legal action against a number of dietary supplement promoters or Web sites that promote or sell dietary supplements because they have made false or deceptive statements about their products or because marketed products have proven to be unsafe.

Sources of Science-Based Information

It's important to look for reliable sources of information on dietary supplements so you can evaluate the claims that are made about them. The most reliable information on dietary supplements is based on the results of rigorous scientific testing.

To get reliable information on a particular dietary supplement:

- Ask your health care providers. Even if they do not know about a specific dietary supplement, they may be able to access the latest medical guidance about its uses and risks.
- Look for scientific research findings on the dietary supplement. The National Center for Complementary and Alternative Medicine (NCCAM) and the National Institutes of Health (NIH) Office of Dietary Supplements (ODS), as well as other Federal agencies, have free publications, clearinghouses, and information on their Web sites.

Safety Considerations

If you are thinking about or are using a dietary supplement, here are some points to keep in mind.

Tell your health care providers about any complementary and alternative practices you use, including dietary supplements. Give them a full picture of what you do to manage your health. This will help ensure coordinated and safe care. (For tips about talking with your health care providers about complementary and alternative medicine (CAM), see NCCAM's Time to Talk campaign at nccam.nih.gov/timetotalk/.) It is especially important to talk to your health care provider if you are

- Thinking about replacing your regular medication with one or more dietary supplements.
- Taking any medications (whether prescription or over-the-counter), as some dietary supplements have been found to interact with medications.
- Planning to have surgery. Certain dietary supplements may increase the risk of bleeding or affect the response to anesthesia.
- Pregnant or nursing a baby, or are considering giving a child a dietary supplement. Most dietary supplements have not been tested in pregnant women, nursing mothers, or children.

If you are taking a dietary supplement, **read the label instructions.** Talk to your health care provider if you have any questions, particularly about the best dosage for you to take. If you experience any side effects that concern you, stop taking the dietary supplement, and contact your health care provider. You can also report your experience to the FDA's MedWatch program. Consumer safety reports on dietary supplements are an important source of information for the FDA.

Keep in mind that although many dietary supplements (and some prescription drugs) come from natural sources, **"natural" does not always mean "safe."** For example, the herbs comfrey and kava can cause serious harm to the liver. Also, a manufacturer's use of the term "standardized" (or "verified" or "certified") does not necessarily guarantee product quality or consistency.

Be aware that **an herbal supplement may contain dozens of compounds** and that its active ingredients may not be known. Researchers are studying many of these products in an effort to identify active ingredients and understand their effects in the body. Also consider the possibility that what's on the label may not be what's in the bottle. Analyses of dietary supplements sometimes find differences between labeled and actual ingredients. For example:

- An herbal supplement may not contain the correct plant species.
- The amount of the active ingredient may be lower or higher than the label states. That means you may be taking less—or more—of the dietary supplement than you realize.
- The dietary supplement may be contaminated with other herbs, pesticides, or metals, or even adulterated with unlabeled ingredients such as prescription drugs.

For current information from the Federal Government on the safety of particular dietary supplements, check the "Dietary Supplement Alerts and Safety Information" section of the FDA Web site at *http://www.fda.gov/Food* /DietarySupplements/Alerts/default.htm or the "Alerts and Advisories" section of the NCCAM Web site at nccam.nih.gov/news/.

Dietary Supplements Research at the National Institutes of Health

NCCAM, which is part of NIH, is the Federal Government's lead agency for studying all types of CAM. As part of that role, the Center sponsors a wide array of research to see how dietary supplements might affect the body and tests their use in clinical trials. In fiscal year 2007, NCCAM supported more than 200 research projects studying dietary supplements, including herbs and botanicals.

Also within NIH, ODS focuses specifically on dietary supplements, seeking to strengthen knowledge by supporting and evaluating research, disseminating results, and educating the public.

NCCAM and ODS collaborate to fund dietary supplement research centers focused on botanicals, known collectively as the NIH Botanical Research Centers Program. Scientists at the centers conduct basic research and other studies on botanicals and help to select products to be tested in clinical trials. The centers are advancing the scientific base of knowledge about botanicals, making it possible to better evaluate their safety and effectiveness.

NCCAM also sponsors a number of Centers of Excellence for Research on CAM, including centers studying antioxidant therapies, botanicals for autoimmune and inflammatory diseases, grape-derived polyphenols for Alzheimer's disease, and botanicals for pancreatic diseases and for colorectal cancer.

Selected References

Barnes, P. M., Bloom, B. & Nahin, R. (2008). Complementary and alternative medicine use among adults and children: United States, 2007. *CDC National Health Statistics Report #12*.

Dietary Supplement Health and Education Act of (1994). U.S. Food and Drug

Administration Web site. Accessed at http://www.fda.gov/opacom/laws/dshea.html on May 12, 2008.

Dietary supplements: background information. (2008). Office of Dietary Supplements Web site. Accessed at *http://ods.od.nih.gov/factsheets/Dietary*Supplements_pf.asp on November 18.

Dietary supplements: overview. (2008). U.S. Food and Drug Administration, Center for Food Safety and Applied Nutrition Web site. Accessed at http://www.cfsan.fda.gov/~dms/supplmnt.html on May 12.

Natural Medicines Comprehensive Database. (2008). Product monographs. Accessed at http://www.naturaldatabase.com on May 13.

Radimer, K., Bindewald, B., Hughes, J., et al. (2004). Dietary supplement use by US adults: data from the National Health and Nutrition Examination Survey, 1999-2000. *American Journal of Epidemiology,160*(4), 339-349.

For More Information

NCCAM Clearinghouse

The NCCAM Clearinghouse provides information on CAM and NCCAM, including publications and searches of Federal databases of scientific and medical literature. The Clearinghouse does not provide medical advice, treatment recommendations, or referrals to practitioners.

Toll-free in the U.S.: 1-888-644-6226
TTY (for deaf and hard-of-hearing callers): 1-866-464-3615
Web site: nccam.nih.gov
E-mail: info@nccam.nih.gov

Office of Dietary Supplements (ODS)

ODS seeks to strengthen knowledge and understanding of dietary supplements by evaluating scientific information, supporting research, sharing research results, and educating the public. Its resources include publications (such as *What Dietary Supplements Are You Taking?*), fact sheets on a variety of specific supplement ingredients (such as vitamin D and black cohosh), and the International Bibliographic Information on Dietary Supplements (IBIDS) database.

Web site: www.ods.od.nih.gov

E-mail: ods@nih.gov

U.S. Food and Drug Administration (FDA)

The FDA oversees the safety of many products, such as foods, medicines, dietary supplements, medical devices, and cosmetics. Its series of consumer updates includes the publication *FDA 101: Dietary Supplements* (*www.fda.gov/downloads*/ForConsumers/ConsumerUpdates/ucm050824.pdf).

Web site: www.fda.gov

Toll-free in the U.S.: 1-888-463-6332

Center for Food Safety and Applied Nutrition (CFSAN)

CFSAN oversees the safety and labeling of supplements, foods, and cosmetics. Online resources for consumers include "Tips for the Savvy Supplement User: Making Informed Decisions and Evaluating Information" and dietary supplement safety alerts.

Web site: www.fda.gov/AboutFDA/CentersOffices/CFSAN/default.htm

Toll-free in the U.S.: 1–888–723–3366

MedWatch

MedWatch, the FDA's safety information and adverse event reporting program, allows consumers and health care providers to file reports on serious problems suspected with dietary supplements.

Web site: www.fda.gov/Safety/MedWatch/HowToReport/ucm053074.htm

Toll-free in the U.S.: 1–888–463–6332

Federal Trade Commission (FTC)

The FTC is the Federal agency charged with protecting the public against unfair and deceptive business practices. A key area of its work is the regulation of advertising (except for prescription drugs and medical devices).

Web site: www.ftc.gov

Toll-free in the U.S.: 1-877-382-4357

PubMed®

A service of the National Library of Medicine (NLM), PubMed contains publication information and (in most cases) brief summaries of articles from scientific and medical journals. CAM on PubMed, developed jointly by NCCAM and NLM, is a subset of the PubMed system and focuses on the topic of CAM.

Web site: www.ncbi.nlm.nih.gov/sites/entrez

CAM on PubMed: nccam.nih.gov/research/camonpubmed/

National Library of Medicine's MedlinePlus and Dietary Supplements Labels Database

To provide resources that help answer health questions, MedlinePlus brings together authoritative information from the National Institutes of Health as well as other Government agencies and health-related organizations.

Web site: www.medlineplus.gov

The Dietary Supplements Labels Database provides information about ingredients in more than 2,000 selected brands of dietary supplements, including vitamins, minerals, herbs or other botanicals, amino acids, and other specialty supplements.

Web site: http://dietarysupplements.nlm.nih.gov/dietary/

CHAPTER SOURCES

The following chapters have been previously published:

Chapter 1 – These remarks were delivered as Statement of Senator Herb Kohl, before the Special Committee on Aging Hearing, given May 26, 2010.

Chapter 2 – This is an edited, excerpted and augmented edition of a United States Government Accountability Office publication, Report Order Code GAO-10-662T, dated May 26, 2010.

Chapter 3 – These remarks were delivered as Statement of Tod Cooperman, MD, before the Special Committee on Aging Hearing, given May 26, 2010.

Chapter 4 – These remarks were delivered as Statement of Charles Bell, before the Special Committee on Aging Hearing, given May 26, 2010.

Chapter 5 – These remarks were delivered as Statement of Steve Mister, before the Special Committee on Aging Hearing, given May 26, 2010.

Chapter 6 – These remarks were delivered as Statement of Joshua M. Sharfstein MD, before the Special Committee on Aging Hearing, given May 26, 2010.

Chapter 7 – This is an edited, excerpted and augmented edition of a National Institute on Aging publication.

Chapter 8 – This is an edited, excerpted and augmented edition of a United StatesFood and Drug Administration publication, dated August 4, 2008.

Chapter 9 – This is an edited, excerpted and augmented edition of a United States Department of Health and Human Services publication.

INDEX

D

E

F